Achieving **Antiracism** in **Medical Education**

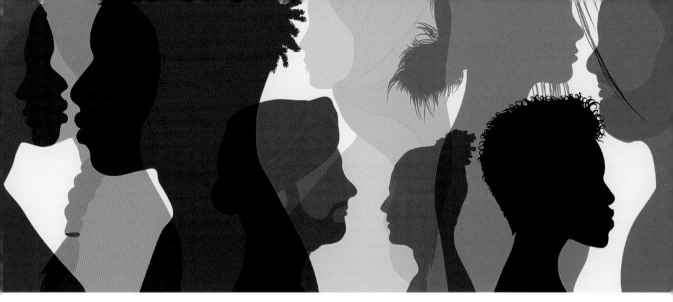

Achieving **Antiracism** in **Medical Education**

Transforming the Culture

LEONA HESS, PhD
Co-Director, Institute for Equity and Justice in Health
    Sciences Education
Icahn School of Medicine at Mount Sinai
New York, New York

ANN-GEL PALERMO, DrPH, MPH
Associate Professor, Leni and Peter May Department of
    Medical Education
Senior Associate Dean for Diversity, Equity, and Inclusion
Icahn School of Medicine at Mount Sinai
Chief Diversity, Equity, and Inclusion Officer in
    Education and Research
Office for Diversity and Inclusion
Mount Sinai Health System
New York, New York

DAVID MULLER, MD
Director, Institute for Equity and Justice in Health
    Sciences Education
Dean Emeritus, Medical Education
Professor of Medical Education and Medicine
Icahn School of Medicine at Mount Sinai
New York, New York

ELSEVIER

Elsevier
1600 John F. Kennedy Blvd.
Ste 1800
Philadelphia, PA 19103-2899

ACHIEVING ANTIRACISM IN MEDICAL EDUCATION   ISBN: 978-0-443-11291-1

Notice

Practitioners and researchers must always rely on their own experience and knowledge in evaluating and using any information, methods, compounds or experiments described herein. Because of rapid advances in the medical sciences, in particular, independent verification of diagnoses and drug dosages should be made. To the fullest extent of the law, no responsibility is assumed by Elsevier, authors, editors or contributors for any injury and/or damage to persons or property as a matter of products liability, negligence or otherwise, or from any use or operation of any methods, products, instructions, or ideas contained in the material herein.

The opinions expressed in this book are the author's opinions and do not necessarily reflect the views of Icahn School of Medicine at Mount Sinai or the Mount Sinai Health System.

Any anecdotes or stories shared are either hypothetical or a reflection of what the authors learned from their work with other medical schools in North America, and these examples or discussions of school operations are not grounded in the authors' work at Mount Sinai except where specifically noted.

Content Strategist: Elyse O'Grady
Senior Content Development Specialist: Vaishali Singh
Publishing Services Manager: Shereen Jameel
Project Manager: Shereen Jameel
Design Direction: Brian Salisbury

Printed in India

Last digit is the print number: 9 8 7 6 5 4 3 2 1

Working together to grow libraries in developing countries

www.elsevier.com • www.bookaid.org

The seeds of antiracist transformation at Icahn School of Medicine at Mount Sinai were planted in December 2014, when medical students at our school and across the nation staged die-ins to protest the murders of Eric Garner, Michael Brown, and Tamir Rice at the hands of police.

The election of Donald Trump to the presidency in 2017 put all of our work in jeopardy and taught us important lessons in perseverance and resourcefulness. We had no intention of diminishing or suspending our efforts despite the looming threat of his administration.

The COVID pandemic demonstrated once again the stark disparities in morbidity and mortality experienced by communities of color. It also brought to light anti-Asian racism and a shocking rise of violent anti-Asian hate crimes.

An intense national focus on antiracism and racial justice was born in the wake of the murders of Breonna Taylor, Ahmaud Arbery, and George Floyd in 2020. This resurgence brought with it resources, rhetoric, and a rejuvenation of efforts to combat racism in all its forms.

In 2023, the Supreme Court of the United States (SCOTUS) handed down decisions that began dismantling protections and liberties that have been the bedrock of this nation's aspirations for all its citizens. In the wake of these rulings, anti-DEI resources, rhetoric, and action are on the rise.

Most recently, since the terrorist attack on October 7, 2023 and the subsequent war in Gaza, there has been a shocking increase in instances of antisemitic and Islamophobic hate speech and hate crimes, in particular at institutions of higher education.

One might say that in the setting of these historic events our timing in writing this book was perfect, but that would be missing the point. Antiracism is never without chaos and crisis. Our own efforts at Icahn School of Medicine are punctuated by these events, as is this nation's history of race relations and oppression. It is entirely predictable that we will recover, albeit slowly and incompletely, from these experiences, only to suffer further setbacks in the coming years.

While crisis and chaos are most prominent on a national scale, there is no shortage of examples that happen regionally, institutionally, within departments, and even among colleagues. Changes in leadership or in "strategic priorities," budgetary constraints, accreditation cycles, and resistance to change can all contribute to episodic crises that can derail efforts at achieving racial justice. These and many other events have disrupted our efforts at antiracism and the efforts of our colleagues.

Moments of crisis and chaos can lead to societal breakdowns and feelings that include rage, fear, and hopelessness. Conversely, the breakdowns we experience can become breakthroughs thanks to the courage, creativity, and relentless efforts of people who are willing to challenge the status quo, often putting their futures, and sometimes even their lives, on the line. In medical education these are our students, residents, and junior faculty, and in each of these groups it is disproportionately people of color who bear the burden of this work.

This breakdown/breakthrough cycle is the key to transformational change and is the reason we began our journey. Sustaining and nourishing the breakthroughs is the reason we wrote this book. Writing this book has allowed us to think critically about our own experiences with antiracism, as well as our effort to disseminate our model to other medical schools in North America through Anti-Racist Transformation in Medical Education, a program generously funded by the Josiah Macy, Jr. Foundation. The exercise of "putting pen to paper" has helped us refine an approach that we believe can be profoundly impactful.

This book is intended to be used as a guide for institutions that are hoping to dig deeper and achieve staying power in their antiracism; something with which we struggled for decades before learning about transformational change. Unlike other books, this is not a how-to-be-antiracist training manual. Every institution, indeed, every individual, will have to figure that out for themselves in the setting of their culture, values, resources, and lived experience. What this book does offer is an approach to developing the capacity for change: establishing a strong and lasting foundation that will maximize the likelihood that antiracism will remain firmly in place long after all of us have moved on.

There is no doubt that institutions and individual people will continue to undo, undermine, and otherwise disrupt efforts at addressing racism and bias. Our hope is that the lessons learned from this book will help our readers anticipate these crises, harness the chaos, and course correct in a manner that makes it clear; we may have lost a battle, but we continue to win the war. This steadfast belief is what allowed Dr. Martin Luther King, Jr. to quote 19th century abolitionist and Unitarian minister Theodore Parker when he said that "the arc of the moral universe is long, but it bends towards justice."

What Do We Mean by "Antiracism"?

Language evolves as our appreciation for and understanding of the world around us evolves. This is especially true for language that describes major social movements, and the term antiracism is no exception.

We believe that it is important to offer our definition of antiracism and some context for that definition so that we can best articulate our intentions, goals, and aspirations.

Context

In the 16th and 17th centuries the concept of race established a social hierarchy where people of color were considered inferior in every way to people who were White. In the Americas anti-black racism was used to justify slavery and anti-indigenous racism was used to justify colonization. (https://nmaahc.si.edu/learn/talking-about-race/topics/historical-foundations-race.)

National Museum of African American History & Culture (Smithsonian)

In the United States, once this social hierarchy was established it was easy to apply it to other groups who were taken advantage of and mistreated – including Mexican, Chinese, Irish, Italian, Jewish, Muslim, and Puerto Rican people.

As a result, anti-black and anti-indigenous racism have always been at the core when it comes to other forms of bias. While we denounce all phobias and –isms, we know that any effort to eliminate them requires an unflinching focus on their root cause. By centering our efforts on those who have been most marginalized in our society, we enable ourselves to better understand, empathize with, and eventually eliminate systems of oppression that affect us all. That is the nature of the '+' in our coining the term "Antiracism+". This is especially true today, as the nation is experiencing a surge in antisemitism and Islamophobia, much of which is coming to a head on college campuses.

What Does It Mean?

Antiracism does not focus exclusively on people who are Black and/or Indigenous. In addition, centering Black and Indigenous voices is not a zero-sum endeavor. Like other holistic ideals (love, empathy, respect, collaboration), the more antiracist we strive to be the more we amplify the positive impact on all other marginalized groups.

The effort to become antiracist explicitly encompasses all other forms of oppression.

Antiracism requires that we accept two core obligations: 1) establishing an environment that allows everyone, especially people from marginalized communities, to achieve their full potential; 2) always being vigilant to, and acting on, manifestations of racism/bias in one's environment.

What Does It Look Like?

In this book we have included antiracist practices at the start of each chapter. You may be surprised to learn that these practices have nothing to do with racism per se. In fact they read very much like sage advice from the very best literature on leadership skills and team-building. Yet they have everything to do with creating a culture that will not tolerate racism or any form of bias. These practices are Critical Self-Reflection; Accountability; Power-Sharing; Naming the Discomfort; and Micro-affirmations.

Why Is This Important to Us?

Medical education and the medical profession have played a significant role in establishing and reinforcing a racial social hierarchy over the course of centuries. Examples include experimenting on Black, Brown, and Indigenous people;[1] perpetuating pseudo-scientific beliefs about Black, Brown, and Indigenous peoples' bodies;[2,3] allowing segregated care and disparities in health outcomes to persist; and teaching scientific racism.[4] Many of these issues continue to linger and demand urgent attention if we are to set an example for a society of justice, equity, and human rights as core principles of medical education, biomedical research, and clinical practice.

The Best Way to Use This Book?

While this methodology was developed at a medical school to address racism and bias, at its core it is a change management strategy that can be harnessed to transform the culture at any health sciences education school. We continue to work with our colleagues in nursing, social work, and physical therapy schools among others.

We have also harnessed this approach to address ALL forms of bias at our school, whether it be related to race, gender, religion, sexual orientation/gender identity, disability, or others. This has always been our priority and has taken on increasing importance at different moments in history: for example, anti-Asian bias at the height of the COVID pandemic and the recent spike in antisemitism and Islamophobia as a result of terrorist attacks and the war in the Middle East.

This book introduces concepts and different ways of thinking, exercises, case examples, and resource materials to help develop the capacity of individuals and institutions. It provides examples and anecdotes that hopefully resonate with your own experiences and is interspersed with what we call "Wicked" questions that are meant to be probing and thought provoking.

- *Do the exercises.* If you are unfamiliar with engaging in group exercises, it might feel uncomfortable. Be mindful of the ways in which your discomfort could influence you to rush through the exercises or prevent you from engaging deeply. The exercises pose Wicked questions to help you investigate what you know and the process towards transformation.

- *Take time.* Choose a pace that works for you and/or your team. Going too quickly through the content and exercises often results in missing some of the most useful and transformative experiences. It is fine if you need to revisit a concept, exercise, or case example. You will not find a linear path to an antiracist future in a few days, weeks, or months. Give yourself the gift of time. We invite you to disrupt the sense of urgency.

- *Realize that people are at different stages of readiness.* The goal is not to get everyone to be at the same stage and marching in lockstep. Use the book as a roadmap and an opportunity to align people to the process, with permission to course correct when needed.

REFERENCES

1. Washington H. *Medical Apartheid: The Dark History of Medical Experimentation on Black Americans from Colonial Times to the Present.* Vintage Publishing; 2008.
2. Roberts DE. *Fatal Invention: How Science, Politics, and Big Business Re-Create Race in the Twenty-First Century.* London: New Press; 2012.
3. Braun L. *Breathing Race into the Machine: The Surprising Career of the Spirometer from Plantation to Genetics.* University of Minnesota Press; 2014.
4. Amutah C, Greenidge K, Mante A, et al. Misrepresenting race - The role of medical schools in propagating physician bias. *N Engl J Med.* 2021;384(9):872-878. doi:10.1056/NEJMms2025768.

ACKNOWLEDGMENTS

The ideas, perspectives, strategies, and tools described in this book are the product of many years of collaboration, with input from countless people who have been our teachers, mentors, role models, students, and peers.

More than anyone else, we want to acknowledge the profound impact of students at Icahn School of Medicine at Mount Sinai (ISMMS). They have been a beacon in our journey to be antiracist. They have challenged us, inspired us, shown us the way, and been our willing partners. The Anti-Racism Coalition got us started and set the tone for the level of intense commitment that this work would require.

Our colleagues and peers at ISMMS continue to sustain these antiracism efforts at every level of leadership, across departments, and within their teams. These include the Strategic Leadership Collaborative, which oversees the MD program; the Office of Diversity and Inclusion; and our Guiding Coalition, with its seven spheres: Student Affairs, Curricular Affairs, Admissions, Student Services, School Wide, Student, and Clinical.

A handful of people devoted themselves to envisioning, designing, and implementing Anti-Racist Transformation in Medical Education (ART in Med Ed), out of which grew the idea for this book and the passion for sharing its concepts with a larger audience. This powerful team included Jennifer Dias, Chloe Martin, and Mya Eveland. Jennifer was a medical student who devoted a scholarly year to this project. Brilliant, phenomenally organized, tireless, and brimming with ideas and energy, Jennifer helped bring this work to life and it was through her eyes that we could see the potential impact on generations of teachers and learners. Chloe and Mya worked strategically and diligently to ensure the content development and design was well organized, customized, and engaging. They carefully considered how people learn and what materials and methods will most effectively meet the project aims.

ART in Med Ed gave us the gift of deep relationships with the cohorts of staff and faculty at 11 medical schools in North America: Brody School of Medicine, East Carolina University; the College of Medicine, University of Saskatchewan; Columbia University Vagelos College of Physicians and Surgeons; David Geffen School of Medicine at the University of California, Los Angeles; Duke University School of Medicine; the George Washington University School of Medicine and Health Sciences; the Ohio State University College of Medicine; University of Arizona College of Medicine, Phoenix; University of Minnesota Medical School; University of Missouri-Columbia School of Medicine; and the University of the Incarnate Word School of Osteopathic Medicine. These peers and colleagues taught us much more than we could ever have conveyed to them, and helped us establish an antiracist community of practice that is still going strong. We have the Josiah Macy Jr. Foundation to thank for the grant that made all of this possible.

Anderson and Anderson, Kotter, Prosci, and other change management and transformational change organizations and leaders have provided tools, content, models, frameworks, and inspiration. We could not have developed our process and approach without their groundbreaking contributions.

Our work exists within the larger context and longer historical arc of the revolutionary traditions of antiracism and the more contemporary *antiracism movement* that has been going strong since the 1970s. This movement has its luminaries, its foot soldiers, and everything in between. We are proud to carry on this tradition, and to do our part in folding it into the work of medical education.

Finally, but foremost, we acknowledge the pain, suffering, and loss of life that has sustained this work over hundreds of years. Slavery, lynchings, mass incarceration, and state-sponsored murders by law enforcement are only some of the violence that has been perpetrated on Black and Brown bodies. This chronic and vicious racism has had seminal moments, like the murders of Eric Garner and George Floyd that have ignited movements. We hope and pray that our small efforts contribute to a world that no longer relies on tragedy to sustain itself.

INTRODUCTION

Centuries ago, coinciding with an explosive growth of exploration and colonization, the concept of a hierarchy of races was developed in order to justify political, financial, and social gain. This concept has had remarkable staying power, despite overwhelming evidence that the basis for racial inferiority is not biological or genetic, but is premised on the human desire for power, influence, control, and privilege.

Housing, education, law enforcement, the criminal justice system, and access to healthy food, clean air and water, and medical care have all been influenced by racism and bias.[1] Racism in the United States has also laid the groundwork for other forms of bias, be they based on immigration status, religion, or sexual orientation/gender identity. The willingness to label a group of people as the "other" has its roots in slavery and continues to have profound political, social, and economic consequences, as is evidenced by the fierce decades-long debate about "illegal" immigrants and the recent resurgence of antisemitism.

Medicine has also been shaped by a legacy of racism, permeating clinical practice and biomedical research, health policy, and academic advancement.[2,3] In academic medicine its most profound influence is on medical education, because it is through medical education that the lessons we teach about racism and bias are perpetuated across generations.[4] This includes disparities in medical student recruitment and admissions; inequity in faculty recruitment, retention, and promotion; and the deeply flawed "correction" factors that we continue to teach our students.[5]

In recent years medical schools have begun to tackle this deeply ingrained reality. Most efforts, however, have focused largely on discrete targets such as curricular content, recruitment strategies, and unconscious bias training. These actions fall short of addressing the systems and structures of racism. Because racism influences the culture of medical education – our beliefs, values, and attitudes – dismantling racism in medical schools requires a strategy that is broadly transformative, lifelong, people dependent, and responsive to the world around us.

In this book we describe an approach to becoming and being an antiracist institution. This approach, when compared to the methods and strategies traditionally employed in medical school, is counterintuitive. Progress in academic medicine tends to be task-oriented, time-limited, and output-based, requiring linear thinking and clearly defined end points. We propose an alternative: a naturally winding path that requires broad participation from as wide a swath of constituents as possible, deep reflection, the courage to constantly course correct, the willingness to acknowledge that there can be no time limit because this effort must outlive us, and the honesty to admit that the future desired state is unknowable. All we can hope for is to continue the striving.

In Chapter 1 we explore race and racism, briefly touching on their history and delving more deeply into the levels of racism that have been intricately constructed over time. These levels of racism – internalized, interpersonal, institutional, systemic, and cultural – are like nesting matryoshka dolls, enfolding and reinforcing each other as they serve to sustain the status quo despite centuries of concerted efforts to undo racism.

From there we describe the ways in which the functional areas and missions of an MD educational program can perpetuate longstanding inequities and injustice, while cloaking them in the belief that medical education's policies, processes, evaluations, and rewards are merit based.

Chapter 2, Changing the Water, is an exploration of transformational change and its relationship to antiracism. How does one achieve true and lasting cultural transformation related to something as deeply ingrained as racism? The strategy we propose takes a *systems change* approach, implementing change management that is institutionally transformational and individually transformative. We link this to antiracism, a philosophy that demands cross-cutting conscious efforts and deliberate actions to achieve racial equity and racial justice.

The remaining chapters are essentially a how-to manual, devoted to describing our Change Process Roadmap in detail. We provide the reader with a practical, step-by-step, hands-on approach that can be tailored to any institution's circumstances, regardless of existing culture, resources, and current commitment to antiracism or any other form of bias.

We begin with Phase 1: Assessing Readiness for Change. A cohort of faculty, staff and students will cocreate a brave space that will allow them to assess their individual and institutional readiness for change, and ultimately gauge the capacity of a small cohort of faculty, staff, and students to lead the change.

Phase 2: Preparing for Change, is the next step in this process. Cohort members clarify their roles, establish optimal working relationships, and identify a project (or target) community. The cohort may choose to focus on a particular department or program, or be more ambitious and cast a wider net in identifying the community within which they hope to achieve the transformational change. Once the *project community* has been identified, the cohort will clarify the case for change, which includes determining the initial desired outcome.

Now that the overall change strategy has been clarified, it is time for Phase 3: Creating a Climate for Change. The cohort will build an understanding of the case for change among members of its project community by generating a sense of urgency, role modeling a commitment to change, and building a powerful, enthusiastic group of change leaders called a *Guiding Coalition*. This Guiding Coalition will develop a set of values and core principles that will guide its work, begin the work of creating an infrastructure to support the change, and "take the show on the road" by communicating the vision, strategy, and process for change to its project community members.

In Phase 4, Engaging and Enabling the Institution for Change, the Guiding Coalition will develop its first set of 1-year *change targets*, tactical plans for achieving those targets, and methods for monitoring outcomes and performance. The Coalition will also establish strategies for integration and acceleration that will empower and sustain broad-based action, ultimately generating short-term wins and enabling clear and consistent communication with all stakeholders.

"Phase Five" is actually a misnomer. Instead of a separate phase, it actually describes the steps the Guiding Coalition will take to ensure that the foundation that has been established becomes a lifelong and self-sustaining cycle. The initial wave of change targets will

be implemented and become an annual exercise. Along the way, the Guiding Coalition and others in the project community will support integration and mastery of change management into the work and learning environments. The importance of celebrating achievements will be recognized and formalized as part of this ongoing cycle, as will the process of anticipating, identifying, and removing barriers to change. More than anything else this is meant to be a learning cycle, recognizing that we often learn the most when we fall short and course correct.

In the final sections of the book we address the infrastructure and support needed to stand up and sustain these efforts. This includes defining the leadership and influencer roles that are critical to the process, and the ways in which the cohort and Guiding Coalition can liaise and collaborate with other entities working on shared goals. We also discuss the importance of establishing or joining an interinstitutional *antiracist medical education community of practice*, which has the potential to offer shared experiences and knowledge, as well as best practices.

In the last section of the book we offer various examples of programs and initiatives that our school has launched and sustained as a result of our transformational change. Many of these outcomes are student centric, such as student leadership opportunities, antiracism fellowships, and funded scholarly years. Others, such as learning labs, are focused on staff, ensuring that voices of these often-neglected yet critically important members of our community are uplifted and contribute to the change. We also describe in detail our curriculum clinics, a series of faculty-focused foundational workshops, faculty development opportunities, assessment tools, and coaching sessions that help create inclusive learning environments and prepare educators to identify and mitigate racism and bias.

REFERENCES

1. Human Rights Watch. Racial *Discrimination in the United States: Human Rights Watch/ACLU Joint Submission Regarding the United States' Record Under the International Convention on the Elimination of All Forms of Racial Discrimination.* Human Rights Watch; Published August 8, 2022. https://www.hrw.org/report/2022/08/08/racial-discrimination-united-states/human-rights-watch/aclu-joint-submission

2. Washington HA. *Medical Apartheid: The Dark History of Medical Experimentation on Black Americans from Colonial Times to the Present*. Paw Prints; 2006.

3. Roberts DE. *Fatal Invention: How Science, Politics, and Big Business Re-Create Race in the Twenty-First Century*. London: New Press; 2012.

4. Amutah C, Greenidge K, Mante A, et al. Misrepresenting race - The role of medical schools in propagating physician bias. *N Engl J Med*. 2021;384(9):872-878. doi:10.1056/NEJMms2025768.

5. Yousif H, Ayogu N, Bell T. The path forward - an antiracist approach to academic medicine. *N Engl J Med*. 2020;383(15):e91. doi:10.1056/NEJMpv2024535.

CONTENTS

The Water We Swim In

RACE AND RACISM

A significant body of literature has been written on race and racism in the United States. In this section we offer an abbreviated discussion on how these concepts manifest as organizing principles of advantage and disadvantage in the United States.

Race is the most profound organizing principle in American Society.[1] When it was first described in the late 17th century, it was not as a result of a new understanding of biology. It was conceived as a framework for organizing and prioritizing social and economic advantage, developed by a predominantly White society based on the preconceived notion that people with lighter or white skin were superior to people with darker or black skin. This framework has permeated American society, including but not limited to housing, employment, education, transportation, and health care.[2] It has also laid the foundation for the treatment of other minority groups, including people who are indigenous to this continent, successive waves of immigrant groups, and religious minorities. We believe that in the United States racism can be considered the tip of the spear, if that spear represents all forms of bias.

Racism can be defined as the act of imposing the values, beliefs, and norms of that predominantly White society on Black and Brown members of society, with neither their input nor their consent. Throughout the history of the United States this has been accomplished explicitly by oppressing, excluding, and silencing the minority group. Preserving power for the dominant group has also been accomplished implicitly by putting requirements, expectations, and rewards in place that are more familiar to the majority group and therefore easier for that group's members to achieve, generation after generation.[3] This dominance has impacted minority groups regardless of their race, country of origin, religion, gender, etc.

To be racist means to perpetuate, often unknowingly, these systems and preferences[1]. All of us accept them on some level. Perpetrators of racial bias do not have to harbor ill will towards people of color[4]. Being racist is just as much an error of omission—failure on our part to think, feel, and act differently—as it is an error of commission.

The antidote to racism is the willingness to constantly question oneself, and the courage to challenge, and often reject conventional wisdom.[5]

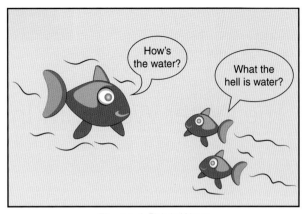

Fig. 1.1 A Fish In Water

A Fish in Water

We are all familiar with the expression "a fish out of water": someone who is awkward, and unfamiliar with their surroundings. What lies at the heart of that expression is an appreciation for what it means to be "a fish in water" (Fig. 1.1). While a fish in water is familiar with its surroundings, it is oblivious to the fact that it is actually swimming in water. For the fish, water is the natural

order of things, allowing it to take entirely for granted that the water even exists.

We find this to be immensely helpful in appreciating the profound impact that racism has on our daily lives, and the role that culture plays in sustaining it. Culture in general is something we typically take for granted. As Tema Okun writes, "culture is so powerful precisely because it is so present and at the same time so difficult to name or identify."[6] Culture is the water we swim in and it has always been polluted by the forces of racism (Fig. 1.1).[7]

The ideology of advantage and disadvantage, superiority and inferiority based on skin color, quite literally "colors" American society: politics, the economy, employment, education, housing, crime, law enforcement, health care, and science.[8,9] Race and racism influence whom we marry and with whom we socialize; where we live; where and with whom we work; how we vote; what we value; where we will send our children to school; how we define good and bad, normal, and abnormal; and who we believe is worthy of resources and support.

As demonstrated in Fig. 1.2, this is true at multiple levels.[10]

Some Americans who are Black, Indigenous, People of Color (BIPOC) *internalize* racist beliefs about their

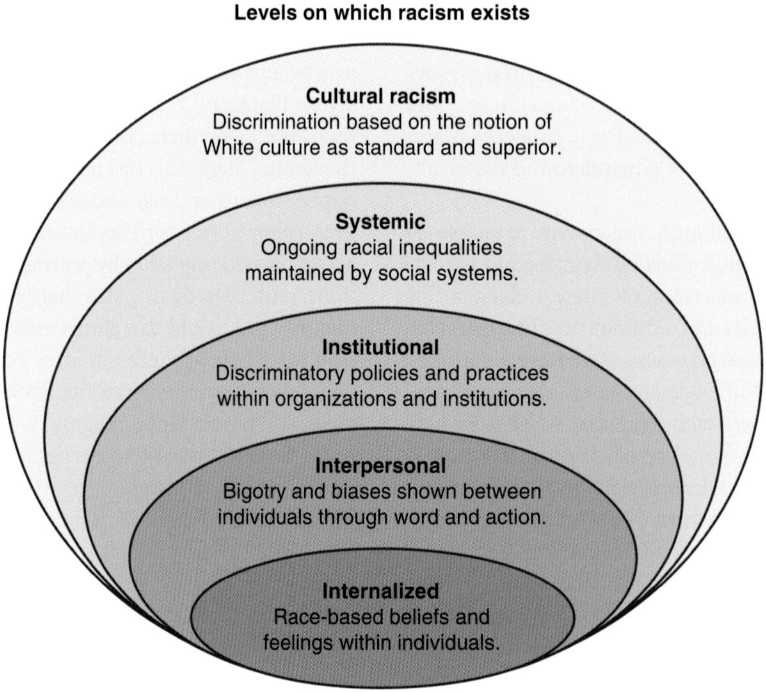

Levels on which racism exists

Cultural racism
Discrimination based on the notion of White culture as standard and superior.

Systemic
Ongoing racial inequalities maintained by social systems.

Institutional
Discriminatory policies and practices within organizations and institutions.

Interpersonal
Bigotry and biases shown between individuals through word and action.

Internalized
Race-based beliefs and feelings within individuals.

Fig. 1.2 Levels on Which Racism Exists

own inferiority and believe that they are destined to be underachievers, not deserving of the same benefits and privilege as many White Americans.

Americans who are BIPOC often experience *interpersonal* racism on a daily basis, some of which is passive (not socializing with one's Black and Brown neighbors), some of which is active (preventing people of color from buying a house in one's neighborhood by not listing it publicly), and some of which is violent (defacing and vandalizing the homes of Black and Brown people in one's neighborhood).

Institutional racism is the practice of establishing, and accumulating over time, rules and policies that unintentionally, and sometimes intentionally, give one group clear advantages over another group.[10] If we were to make the case of institutional advantage using socioeconomic status instead of race, few would deny its existence and profound impact.

And yet when it comes to race we are skeptical, and question whether institutional racism actually exists or is a figment of the imagination, an attempt on the part of people of color to explain away their inability to compete with their White peers. Despite this disbelief, the evidence is abundant. Institutional racism includes racial profiling by law enforcement;[11] racist sentencing policies by the criminal justice system;[1] discriminatory housing and lending policies;[12] political disenfranchisement through voter suppression and gerrymandering;[13] and inadequate funding for education that disproportionately impacts communities of color, in part by being linked to revenue from property taxes and redistricting practices.[12]

Systemic racism is closely tied to, and overlaps with, institutional racism. The policies, procedures, and practices that constitute institutional racism drive persistent and pervasive ("systemic") disparities that perpetuate the perception that people of color are not as capable, not as smart, and not as hard working as their White peers. These beliefs are self-fulfilling, convincing many White people that people of color are not deserving, would disappoint and fail if given an opportunity, and have the potential for ruining the social structures—neighborhoods, schools, jobs—that many White people enjoy.[3] These beliefs also create a positive feedback loop with internalized racism, leaving many people of color feeling bereft, insecure, and unworthy.[14]

These reinforcing levels of racism create a culture in which we are all led to inherently believe that White is not just the norm or the standard, but is actually superior and is the ideal to which we should all strive. This *cultural racism* justifies what we then take to be the natural order: prisons that are filled with Black men, public housing and public schools that are populated by families and children of color, and social services disproportionately being utilized by those very same communities.

RACISM AND MEDICAL EDUCATION

Is medical education racist? In this section we discuss the ways in which racism manifests in medical education, with a specific focus on four key functional areas: curricular affairs, admissions, student affairs, and diversity affairs. Each area of focus concludes with a wicked question for additional reflection.

Consider the following examples, which may be familiar anecdotes at schools across the country. A Black medical student entering the hospital is stopped by a security officer while his White peers pass by; a Latinx medical student complains of racist comments made in the operating room; an Asian medical student submits a mistreatment report describing stereotyping and disrespectful behavior on the part of her residents that she believes was related to her race; a South Asian medical student reports to the Office of Curricular Affairs that a lecturer in the dermatology course stated "normal skin is pale skin" as a teaching point thereby othering patients (and learners) of color. These and similar instances are often dismissed as "not racist": the people being reported did not harbor any ill will towards people of color. In fact they feel terrible that what they thought was a benign comment or "just doing my job" was perceived as racist.

How do we bridge the divide between the lived experience of BIPOC medical students, staff, and faculty that racism is ubiquitous, like the water we swim in, and the belief of so many White people that these claims are exaggerated or simply untrue? Language matters, and an important step is in agreeing on the definition of terms like "racism" and "racist."

Ibram Kendi wrote that:

"One either believes problems are rooted in groups of people, as a racist, or locates the roots of problems in power and policies, as an anti-racist. One either allows racial inequities to persevere, as a racist, or

confronts racial inequities, as an anti-racist. There is no in-between safe space of 'not racist'."[5]

There is extensive evidence demonstrating that BIPOC individuals in the health professions experience disparities when it comes to entry into the health professions, advancement, mentorship, research funding, recruitment and retention, and access to role models.[15–20] As Kendi writes, instead of locating the roots of these problems in people, what is required is locating them in policies and power dynamics that produce inequities for particular groups across race, gender, class, and other intersecting social identities, while providing advantages and benefits to members of the already-privileged dominant group.

Curricular Affairs

A medical school curriculum lays the foundation for what future physicians know to be "the truth" about how the body functions, what happens when things go wrong, and what to do about it when that occurs. It also encompasses the skills, attitudes, and behaviors that are expected of physicians: communication; the physical exam; embracing and respecting difference, and appreciating how that difference impacts health and illness; the social mission of medicine; and much more.

While the teaching of skills, attitudes, and behaviors has begun to incorporate racism, bias, and the impact of social determinants,[21] the bulk of a curriculum and the bulk of what is assessed on examinations constitutes the core of what students will focus on, and where they will devote their efforts. This content continues to revolve around the biomedical model, and by extension, its underpinnings in scientific racism.[22–24]

The *biomedical model* has been the predominant model of illness since the 19th century. Among its core tenets are that: illness results exclusively from biological disruptions within the body, to the exclusion of psychological, social, and environmental influences; health is the absence of disease; and patients are victims of circumstance (Box 1.1).[25] As Tsai and colleagues write, the biomedical model decontextualizes the patient, thereby erasing individual patient perspectives and casting race and sex as simple characteristics and risk factors inherent to individual physiology.[26] It also powerfully reinforces and socializes *scientific racism:* the notion that Black people are not just biologically and/or genetically different, but inferior, and at least partly responsible for

BOX 1.1	Characteristics of Biomedical Model
Concept	**Biomedical Model**
Conceptual basis	Reductionist, mechanistic, inflexible
Application of scientific methods	Relies on objective physical measures, single brief interventions, and randomized controlled trials
Etiology	Pathophysiological etiology based on a single static etiology (e.g., infectious agent, structural change, cancer)
Problem list	Identify chief complaint and diagnosis in the physical or psychiatric realm
Treatment strategy	Unidimensional that encourages single sequential treatments
Providers	Single clinician providing single intervention that is easy to implement may lead to fragmented approaches

Fricton J, Anderson K, Clavel A, et al. Preventing chronic pain: a human systems approach—results from a massive open online course. *Glob Adv Health Med.* 2015;4(5):23-32. doi:10.7453/gahmj.2015.048.

their poorer health outcomes when compared to Whites. Existing "clinical correction factors" that adjust for this biological inferiority abound, and race is used as a biological distinction that explains epidemiologic differences in many illnesses.[27]

Curricular affairs does not just account for what we teach. It includes the critically important questions of who is doing the teaching, how the teaching is accomplished, and how performance is assessed and graded.

In the wake of George Floyd's murder, schools across the country have struggled to address these issues. Race-based science is often handed down without questioning the conventional wisdom physicians and scientists have been taught. Teaching faculty rarely have the opportunity to "unlearn" much of what they know, and reconsider how racism and bias have led to fundamentally flawed science.[27,28] Some faculty continue to struggle with the concept that race is, after all, a social construct, and fail to appreciate that man-made racism is the driving force behind what they have always believed is genetically/biologically hardwired, due to the social and educational failures of people of color, or both.[29]

WICKED QUESTION

Science is constantly evolving, new discoveries are always being made, and radical departures from revered scientific theories are enthusiastically embraced. The body of knowledge defining race as a social construct was established generations ago and is readily available in the literature. Yet there remains substantial resistance to this departure from revered biomedical norms. What are we protecting/preserving? What are we afraid of?

Admissions and Recruitment

Despite concerted efforts at holistically recruiting students who are underrepresented in medicine, the number of Black men entering medical school has actually declined, from 3.1% of the national medical student body in 1978, to 2.9% in 2019.[30] A system that cannot achieve meaningful gains over 40 years despite federal funding, philanthropy, pathway programs addressing every level of education, and countless people working tirelessly to ameliorate this national crisis illustrates the profound complexity of the problem and the countless ways in which that system does not function well.

Among the many variables that collude to maintain a chokehold on aspiring BIPOC students are poor public school education, poor nutrition, a paucity of after-school programs and extracurricular activities, teachers and other authority figures telling Black and Brown children that they are not up to the challenge, financial barriers and the looming nightmare of educational debt, courses like organic chemistry that are intended to weed out all students and disproportionately weed out Black and Brown students, and a lack of privilege in the form of personal and family access to readily available research and shadowing experiences.[15] It is no wonder that impostor syndrome and internalized racism are the natural outcomes of this process.

In fact, many accept this outcome as the norm and continue to consider entrance to medical school as another shining example of American meritocracy.[31]

WICKED QUESTION

Would we accept declining admissions rates for any other identity groups—or would we demand immediate action and tangible results? What is the mindset or deeply held belief that allows us to accept this outcome in the case of Black men?

Student Affairs

Supporting students throughout their journey in medical school, advising and coaching them, paying attention to their academic and personal needs, and distinguishing between the social determinants, social risks, and social needs of their education is a monumental task. Students enter medical school from vastly different backgrounds: from environments of extreme privilege and literally unlimited resources, to lived experiences that include homelessness, food insecurity, and family members who are struggling with incarceration, addiction, and violence.

We find it useful to apply the rubric of social determinants, social risk factors, and social needs to education, in a manner similar to their application to health.[32]

Social *determinants* are underlying structural factors that are not inherently positive or negative. They include state and federal policies that impact housing, education, employment, and social security. They shape health and education for better or worse. They can also be taken for granted by the large segment of society that benefits from America's dominant culture.

Social *risk factors* are always detrimental social conditions that negatively impact health and education. These include housing or food instability, individual experiences with racism, and being underinsured.

Social *needs* are influenced by individual preferences, and are often governed by culture, stigma, impostor syndrome, and internalized racism.

A medical student whose family has been impacted by discriminatory policies (determinants) related to public housing and public schools (risk factors) is going to face greater academic, social, and economic challenges in medical school. That student may feel comfortable seeking out school-supported tutors that they could not otherwise afford, but may not feel comfortable making use of the school's food pantry (needs).

Achieving genuine equity under these circumstances requires a disproportionate distribution of resources. Just as not all students require school support to meet their needs for housing and adequate nutrition, one could argue that not all students require school support for board preparation materials, travel stipends for conferences, and living stipends for scholarly gap years.

And that's just the beginning of the complexity. Advisors, coaches, and mentors are plagued with the same conscious and unconscious biases when interacting with students of color. Professionalism is sometimes misconstrued as expectations for "fitting in" to the culture of medicine and may best suit students who look and sound like their faculty and house-staff role models.[33] Students quickly learn that the reasons they were admitted to medical school (e.g., their values, distance traveled, diversity, and devotion to communities in need) are not the factors that will help them achieve success in the residency application process (e.g., grades, publications, clinical honors, and academic honor societies).

Who Cares?

One might wonder why all of this matters. Of course there is the moral imperative and the desire to "do the right thing." One's conscience may be saying that it is not fair to see so many social, economic, and health disparities fall on the backs of Black and Brown people. But if one fundamentally believes that Black and Brown people are different and partly responsible for their fate, it is not that hard to walk away from it all, firm in the belief that the system works and some people just are not up to the challenge. Although it is not polite to say so, maybe that is why so few students of color make it into medical school, why there are so few faculty of color, and why so few people of color attain leadership positions.

There is, however, another possibility, and one that speaks to much larger forces at play.

Racism has been an organizing principle of American history for four centuries: from its roots as a rationale for enslaving millions of people and benefiting from their free labor, to the convenience of having an oppressed group serve as the perfect scapegoat.[7] American people of color, and in particular Black Americans, have been held up as the group that is trying to take advantage of a system they have not been able to navigate, to "get one over" instead of pulling themselves up by their bootstraps and joining the general meritocracy. According the Heather McGhee in The Sum of Us (3), this method of scapegoating has been used as an excuse for denying, ironically, mostly White Americans the resources and support they need to educate their children, secure gainful employment, and live in clean, safe neighborhoods.

According to McGhee, history also bears out that every time Black Americans have advocated, agitated, and protested for rights, the results have benefited all Americans.[3] Similarly, when Black medical students report that they are disproportionately impacted by subjective evaluations on their clerkships, they are advocating for a transparent system of evaluation that will benefit all.

When Black faculty describe the "minority tax" they pay for shouldering the burdens of diversity, equity, and inclusion (D/E/I) work, they are advocating for academic health centers to do away with their reliance on all "unfunded mandates" from teaching to committee work to mentorship.

The answer to "who cares" is *we all must care*, because racism as a form of oppression impacts everyone and denies us all the dignity, equity, and justice we deserve as fellow citizens.

> **WICKED QUESTION**
>
> What stands in the way of providing medical students from diverse disadvantaged backgrounds with the resources they need to succeed? Why are medical schools reluctant to declare this a strategic priority that is equal in importance to research and clinical care?

DIVERSITY AFFAIRS – A PARADOX

The murder of George Floyd launched the Association of American Medical Colleges (AAMC) on a journey to become an antiracist organization. This journey lifted up diversity, equity, and inclusion as core guiding principles and created a desire to learn and adopt antiracist practices and behaviors along the continuum of medical education. As part of this effort, in June 2020 the AAMC released a strategy to address structural racism within its organization, in academic medicine, and beyond.[34]

However, long before the murder of George Floyd, diversity affairs had its place in medical education, albeit one that had been historically undervalued. According to the AAMC, diversity affairs is responsible for positioning diversity, equity, and inclusion as a key driver of educational excellence, a diverse physician workforce, and ultimately equitable health care for all.[35] It has never been seen as a perpetrator of racism in medical education.

The role, scope, and structure of diversity affairs in medical education is not standardized, leading to significant variability in how it is situated and resourced in medical education and within an organization. It is important to note that diversity affairs is not critical to the basic operation of a medical school and as a result does not have positional power or authority over key functional areas such as admissions, curricular affairs, and student affairs. Thus it is no accident that diversity affairs is often marginalized in the medical education landscape, fostering a mindset among leaders that it is at best an "add-on," and at worst a place where problems related to diversity, equity, and inclusion are sent to be "fixed." In turn, the typical response from diversity affairs colleagues is to show up as a "fixer" or "expert" on disrupting racism, perpetuating the mindset described above. The "add-on" mindset is profound, insidious, and contributes to the paradoxical nature of diversity affairs.

The extent to which diversity affairs colleagues are able to disrupt this paradox lies in their ability to effectively influence without authority. This requires a delicate balance of developing expertise in the practice of diversity, equity, and inclusion; developing and nurturing meaningful, trusting relationships with colleagues; and having a thorough understanding of how an institution operates. The first step to disrupting this paradox is to recognize their own role in perpetuating racism and bias when their ability to influence without authority is stifled because of organizational structures and the behaviors of medical education colleagues.

Diversity Affairs × Curricular Affairs

A common practice among curricular affairs colleagues who feel the pressure to address health disparities in the curriculum is to call upon diversity affairs colleagues to do a one-off lecture, leading to a "check the box" learning experience for the students and the school. The recent acknowledgement of the need to go beyond health disparities and teach social determinants of health and structural competency also risks leaning on diversity affairs colleagues to develop and teach this content.

These curricular responses assume diversity affairs colleagues are seasoned content experts when they are typically not. Diversity affairs colleagues are often physicians who work in a D/E/I role as a percentage of their full-time job, and may lac content expertise, fromal training in antiracism pedagogy, learning design practices, facilitation techniques to discuss contemporary social issues in medicine. Further, diversity affairs colleagues are often not equipped with the knowledge of how these content areas intersect with systems of education, care, and research.

Unbeknownst to diversity affairs colleagues, their compliance with these curricular affairs requests may reinforce racism in medical education by delivering substandard education that harms the learning environment, learners, and ultimately patients. This harm may be fortified by the behavior of curricular affairs colleagues whose urgency, defensiveness, and either/or thinking prevent them from confronting their own blind spots when it comes to transforming all of medical education into an antiracist learning journey for faculty, staff, and students.

WICKED QUESTION

What is the mental model of how diversity affairs and curricular affairs relate to one another at your institution? What are the drivers of this dynamic that perpetuate racism in your learning environment?

Diversity Affairs × Admissions

Diversity affairs colleagues are often invited by admissions colleagues to partake in recruitment practices to attract applicants who are underrepresented in medicine (URM). Familiar recruitment practices where this collaboration takes place include hosting a "diversity" open house event, participating in premed pathway programming, or being included as part of a "second look" program. However, we fail to examine the ways in which these common and limited collaborations perpetuate the "add-on" mindset and either/or thinking. For example, diversity affairs colleagues are often not consulted or invited to cocreate the design and execution of recruitment and marketing strategies for the medical school. Admissions colleagues see a role of diversity affairs only in terms of limited collaborations and do not make room for both/and thinking that would allow diversity affairs colleagues, who are also student facing, to contribute to a broader portfolio of work. More insidiously, this risks becoming the status quo because diversity affairs colleagues are either waiting to be asked or do not have psychological safety to propose such a role to their admissions colleagues.

WICKED QUESTION

How do we enhance psychological safety? Does the consultative approach of diversity affairs in the admissions space perpetuate future harm by creating an impression that we care about diversity on the surface, without translating into the experience applicants have with the admissions office and ultimately as a matriculated student?

Diversity Affairs × Student Affairs

While medical school admissions trends have evolved to be more holistic, inclusive, and equitable, the culture, policies, and practices of the student support services environment that is receiving an increasingly diverse student cohort has not kept pace.[36] As a key part of the student affairs ecosystem, a benchmark behavior of diversity affairs is to serve as a trusted resource and advocate for students who may be mistreated, marginalized, or otherwise discriminated against.[35] It is in this role that the paradoxical nature of diversity affairs is most profound. As Grieco and colleagues state in their paper on *Integrated Holistic Student Affairs: A Personalized, Equitable, Student-Centered Approach to Student Affairs,* the sink-or-swim culture in medical education is most detrimental to medical students who are URM and disadvantaged, and who may experience a reactive and deficit-oriented student affairs environment because it threatens their likelihood of thriving and achieving success in medical school.[36] As a stakeholder in this type of student affairs environment, the diversity affairs response is to protect the URM student from the harm of student affairs practices and to ensure the student can "swim" by providing guidance and support on how to navigate medical school successfully. It is in this response where we find the paradox.

The first part of the response fosters a mental model that URM and disadvantaged students always sink, unlike their non-URM student counterparts, and that student affairs is ineffective in providing the unique level and type of support these students need. The diversity affairs office will "protect" these underrepresented students and try to fill their unmet needs, even though this office is not organizationally situated or resourced to do so effectively. Thus student affairs avoids the responsibility of figuring out how to support "sinking" students, and diversity affairs risks becoming the default "dumping ground" for URM and disadvantaged students' issues.

Perfectionism, sense of urgency, either/or thinking, and *only one right way* are deeply embedded in the values and structures that support medical education, and are often perpetuated by many student affairs offices.

This is where the paradox shows up in the second part of the response. Diversity affairs colleagues encourage and guide URM and disadvantaged students to identify with, and when necessary adopt, these norms and characteristics in order to achieve success in medical school, all the while believing that they are serving as an advocate without recognizing they have become perpetrators of this ideology.

> **WICKED QUESTION**
>
> What are some ways in which diversity affairs at your school perpetuates these norms and contributes to the experience of racism in your learning environment?

REFERENCES

1. Alexander M. *The New Jim Crow: Mass Incarceration in the Age of Colorblindness.* New York: New Press; 2010.
2. Kendi IX. *Stamped from the Beginning: The Definitive History of Racist Ideas in America.* New York, NY: Nation Books; 2017.
3. McGhee HC. *The Sum of Us: What Racism Costs Everyone and How We Can Prosper Together.* New York, NY: One World; 2021.
4. Banaji MR, Greenwald AG. *Blindspot: Hidden Biases of Good People.* Bantam Books; 2016.
5. Kendi IX. *How to Be an Antiracist.* New York: One World; 2019.
6. Okun T. *White Supremacy Culture.* White Supremacy Culture; 2021. https://www.whitesupremacyculture.info/.
7. DiAngelo R, Dyson ME. *White Fragility: Why It's So Hard for White People to Talk About Racism.* Boston, Beacon Press; 2018
8. Darity WA, Mullen AK. *From Here to Equality: Reparations for Black Americans in The Twenty-First Century.* The University of North Carolina Press; 2022.
9. Roberts D. Fatal invention. Tantor Audio; 2020.
10. Braveman PA, Arkin E, Proctor D, Kauh T, Holm N. Systemic and structural racism: definitions, examples, health damages, and approaches to dismantling. *Health Affairs.* 2022;41(2):171-178. doi:10.1377/hlthaff.2021.01394.
11. Muhammad KG. *The Condemnation of Blackness: Race, Crime, and The Making of Modern Urban America.* Harvard University Press; 2019.
12. Rothstei R. *The Color of Law: A Forgotten History of How our Government Segregated America.* Liveright Publishing Corporation, a division of W.W. Norton & Company; 2018.
13. Downs J. *Voter Suppression in US Elections.* University of Georgia Press; 2020
14. Wilkerson I. *Caste: The Origins of Our Discontents.* Penguin Books; 2023.
15. Lucey CR, Saguil A. The consequences of structural racism on MCAT scores and medical school admissions: the past is prologue. *Acad Med.* 2020;95(3):351-356. doi:10.1097/acm.0000000000002939.

16. Nunez-Smith M, Ciarleglio MM, Sandoval-Schaefer T, et al. Institutional variation in the promotion of racial/ethnic minority faculty at US medical schools. *Am J Public Health*. 2012;102(5):852-858. doi:10.2105/AJPH.2011.300552.

17. Beech BM, Calles-Escandon J, Hairston KG, Langdon SE, Latham-Sadler BA, Bell RA. Mentoring programs for underrepresented minority faculty in academic medical centers. *Acad Med*. 2013;88(4):541-549. doi:10.1097/acm.0b013e31828589e3.

18. Ginther DK, Schaffer WT, Schnell J, et al. Race, ethnicity, and NIH research awards. *Science*. 2011;333(6045):1015-1019. doi:10.1126/science.1196783.

19. Avakame EF, October TW, Dixon GL. Antiracism in academic medicine: fixing the leaky pipeline of black physicians. *ATS Scholar*. 2021;2(2):193-201. doi:10.34197/ats-scholar.2020-0133PS.

20. Pololi L, Cooper LA, Carr P. Race, disadvantage and faculty experiences in academic medicine. *J Gen Intern Med*. 2010;25(12):1363-1369. doi:10.1007/s11606-010-1478-7.

21. AAMC. *Teaching Hospitals' Commitment to Addressing the Social Determinants of Health*. 2017. https://www.aamc.org/media/19686/download.

22. Opara IN, Riddle-Jones L, Allen N. Modern day drapetomania: calling out scientific racism. *J Gen Intern Med*. 2022;37(1):225-226. doi:10.1007/s11606-021-07163-z.

23. Neblett EW Jr. Racism measurement and influences, variations on scientific racism, and a vision. *Soc Sci Med*. 2023;316:115247. doi:10.1016/j.socscimed.2022.115247.

24. Fuentes A. Systemic racism in science: reactions matter. *Science*. 2023;381(6655):eadj7675. doi:10.1126/science.adj7675.

25. Wade DT, Halligan PW. Do biomedical models of illness make for good healthcare systems? *BMJ*. 2004;329(7479):1398-1401. doi:10.1136/bmj.329.7479.1398.

26. Tsai J, Lindo E, Bridges K. Seeing the window, finding the spider: applying critical race theory to medical education to make up where biomedical models and social determinants of health curricula fall short. *Front Public Health*. 2021;9:653643. doi:10.3389/fpubh.2021.653643.

27. Braun L, Fausto-Sterling A, Fullwiley D, et al. Racial categories in medical practice: how useful are they? *PLoS Med*. 2007;4(9):e271. doi:10.1371/journal.pmed.0040271.

28. Cerdeña JP, Plaisime MV, Tsai J. From race-based to race-conscious medicine: how anti-racist uprisings call us to act. *Lancet*. 2020;396(10257):1125-1128. doi:10.1016/S0140-6736(20)32076-6.

29. Evans M, Williams W, Graves J, Shim R, Tishkoff S. Race in medicine — Genetic variation, social categories, and paths to health equity. *N Engl J Med*. 2021;385(14):e45. doi:10.1056/nejmp2113749.

30. Morris DB, Gruppuso PA, McGee HA, Murillo AL, Grover A, Adashi EY. Diversity of the national medical student body — four decades of inequities. *N Engl J Med*. 2021;384(17):1661-1668. doi:10.1056/nejmsr2028487.

31. Stoll I. Opinion | Medical Schools Bail on Academic Merit and Intellectual Rigor. *WSJ*. https://www.wsj.com/articles/medical-schools-bail-on-academic-merit-and-intellectual-rigor-us-news-rankings-diversity-equity-inclusion-race-students-11675005330.

32. Samuels-Kalow ME, Ciccolo GE, Lin MP, Schoenfeld EM, Camargo CA. The terminology of social emergency medicine: measuring social determinants of health, social risk, and social need. *J Am Coll Emerg Physicians Open*. 2020;1(5):852-856. doi:10.1002/emp2.12191.

33. Maristany D, Hauer KE, Leep Hunderfund AN, et al. The problem and power of professionalism: a critical analysis of medical students' and residents' perspectives and experiences of professionalism. *Acad Med*. 2023;98(11S):S32-S41. doi:10.1097/ACM.0000000000005367.

34. AAMC. *Addressing and Eliminating Racism at the AAMC and Beyond*. https://www.aamc.org/addressing-and-eliminating-racism-aamc-and-beyond.

35. AAMC. *GSA Performance Framework*. https://www.aamc.org/professional-development/affinity-groups/gsa/performance-framework.

36. Grieco CA, Currence P, Teraguchi DH, Monroe A, Palermo AGS. Integrated holistic student affairs: a personalized, equitable, student-centered approach to student affairs. *Acad Med*. 2022;97(10):1441-1446. doi:10.1097/acm.0000000000004757.

2

Changing the Water

ANTIRACISM: A JOURNEY WITH NO DESTINATION

Antiracism has a long and rich history and its definition has evolved over time. From the Dominican friars who defied the Spanish crown in the 16th century and denounced the cruelty to American natives, to the Quakers and the American abolitionist movement, to the Civil Rights movement in the 1960s. Most recently, in his book How To Be Antiracist, Ibram Kendi writes:

> *"One either believes problems are rooted in groups of people, as a racist or locates the roots of problems in power and policies, as an antiracist.*
> *One either allows racial inequities to persevere, as a racist, or confronts racial inequities, as an antiracist."[1]*

According to Kendi, choosing *yes* or *no* to the question "are you racist" misses the point of how racism works. The opposite of racist is not "not racist." It is "antiracist." Being antiracist requires that we engage in a process of self-interrogation, asking how racism manifests in oneself and in the systems with which one engages on a daily basis. What we learn from Kendi's distinction is the notion that there is no neutrality in the struggle to overcome racism.

It is also important to note that we use antiracism as a framework for dismantling all forms of bias. Examples include the tragically disproportionate loss of life in communities of color during the COVID pandemic; the rampant anti-Asian bias that grew out of the pandemic; and the resurgence of antisemitism as well as Islamophobia that we are currently experiencing as a nation. Antiracism does focus on race as its leading edge, while being intentionally inclusive in addressing all forms of oppression.

Whether one considers antiracism as an individual or an organization, it is a journey with no defined end point. Because genuine antiracism has never been achieved, one cannot know what the destination looks like, and given the ever-evolving state of society we can be certain that antiracism is not a fixed state. It is lifelong, constantly in flux, and, in light of the many forms that resistance takes, will always require course correction.

As an organization, antiracism starts with changing culture. This is as true for academic medicine as it is for any other organizational structure. Becoming antiracist requires a deep disruption in the way we think, act, speak, make decisions, wield power and privilege, and define quality or success. The way forward requires that we change the water we all swim in.

Change the Water, not the Fish

Context is the frame of reference for the way people in an organization perceive, act, think and relate to one another.[2] Becoming antiracist requires that we examine racism in internalized, interpersonal, institutional, systemic, and cultural contexts (see Fig. 1.1). By interrogating these contexts we can understand that racism is not made up of isolated individuals acts; it is woven through many of our systems and institutions.

The pivot towards becoming antiracist in medicine and medical education requires systemic change. This pivot involves identifying and shifting the conditions (structures, policies, practices, and mindsets) that hold the problem (racism) in place. It calls for recognizing medicine and medical education as a complex and dynamic system with interdependent parts.

The pivot also requires naming these components, from health care delivery systems, to research and technology sectors, and professional societies. All of these components can potentially propagate deeply held traditions, beliefs, and practices, and indoctrinate students, trainees, physicians, and even patients into upholding racist norms and values.[3-5]

Transforming a culture disrupts, dismantles, and reimagines the status quo. Transformation is bold and courageous. It requires that we commit to generating a new and unknown future state that actively ensures we do not return to the default settings that keep racism in place.

Antiracist Transformation

Antiracist transformation is the pathway to reaching this new future state. It is a change process that moves organizations and leaders beyond momentary allyship and performative measures to deeper actions, commitment, and accountability. Antiracist transformation characterizes medicine and medical education as a complex adaptive system (CAS) that requires unlearning the default response of reactive and linear thinking when addressing racism and bias.[6] It requires letting go of the need to tightly control the process of change and recognizes that the environment within which change is happening is messy, dynamic, and unpredictable. It makes room for emerging needs and opportunities.

Antiracist transformation relies on organizational sponsorship upstream, a design-and-build pathway midstream, and implementation downstream. With this full-stream process in place, change can focus on the content (what needs to change) as well as the mindsets and behaviors (the people side of change).[7] When we embrace antiracist transformation as the way forward, we can commit to a lifelong journey with no fixed destination that involves collectively undoing racism and bias at all levels in medicine and medical education.

MORE LIKE A BEEHIVE THAN A CLOCK

A clock and a beehive each have many interdependent and moving parts. A clock, if it is running and in good repair, generally produces a consistent result from one second to the next: it keeps time day and night, week after week, year after year. A clock is predictable, both in the short term and the long term. By contrast, a beehive is a living, breathing, dynamic system. In a beehive, bees work toward what appears to be a common goal: the survival of the colony. The queen bee does not direct the hive. Instead, the roles of each individual bee collectively direct the hive's ultimate goal and outcome. What will happen minute by minute is fairly predictable, but activity in the hive over time is unpredictable. A beehive is a prime example of a CAS, and it is nothing at all like mechanical clockwork.

Similar to a beehive, we live, work, and learn in a CAS. We belong to different groups that consist of semi-autonomous agents who interact in interdependent ways to produce system-wide patterns, and those patterns then influence the behavior of the agents.[6] If we employ a CAS lens to examine the medical education learning environment, we can identify at least three distinct characteristics that make us more like a beehive than a clock. First, the learning environment consists of a number of agents (e.g., students, staff, administrators, faculty, house staff, C-suite leaders, etc.), each of whom has their roles, relationships, and expectations. These agents make decisions about how to behave, and over time these decisions evolve as the actors respond to events and each other.

This leads us to the second characteristic: agents interact with one another to generate dominant patterns of behavior. For example, consider patterns of competition or innovation. Often these behaviors, perhaps perceived as "the rules of the game," are not explicitly articulated or defined. Instead, we learn these patterns over time. Interactions among agents then lead to the third characteristic, emergence. When this happens, the entire system's behavior goes beyond the simple sum of the behaviors of its parts.

If we want to address racism in medical education's CAS we must be able to "see" the system. Often this is challenging because of our siloed structures, limited lines of sight, and investment (conscious or unconscious) in adapting to and maintaining the status quo.

All systems share key features that can aid in our ability to "see" them more clearly.[8]

- A system is complex, dynamic, alive, and exists in a world of many other systems that affect how it functions. For example, the interactions among functional areas of a medical school, between the school and its hospital system, and the Liaison Committee on Medical Education (LCME). They are interdependent and interconnected.
- A system is not the sum of its parts; it is the product of the interactions of those parts. The performance of a medical school depends on how all of the areas perform together, not how they act individually.
- Outcomes in a system have multiple and mutual causalities.
- Visible and invisible feedback loops are essential building blocks of a system. For example, feedback from students can change the curricular content, student support, or financial aid services. On a staff level, if employees feel valued and respected they are more likely to stay in their role for longer periods of time, reducing turnover and cost, improving staff morale, and increasing student satisfaction.
- Mental models—paradigms, mindsets, beliefs, assumptions, cultural narratives, norms, expectations, or simply perceptions—significantly impact how people behave and perform in a system.
- Systems self-organize and self-correct to resist change.
- The system is not "out there." We and the way we learn and work together are a part of it.

Undertaking the task of enacting change in any CAS is daunting as there are so many moving parts. Thus when thinking about change we must create a process that will help identify the parts, as well as reveal and analyze ways in which they interact, some of which are manifest and some of which are hidden. Often things are not what they seem. Complexity defines the relationships among agents and among the system's structures. We must peel back layers of the onion and consider levels within levels. Causation is often deeply buried and we may be unaware of how a distant activity impacts our own actions—the rule of unintended consequences.

Given all of this, before we can address racism in our CAS we must understand the CAS within which we learn and work. There are real pressures to skip this first step. There is an urgency to fix immediate problems. Even if we give ourselves permission to slow down, it is often difficult to see the forest for the trees because our institutions are so complex, deeply hierarchical, and siloed. There is also the challenge of taking an approach that may run counter to "how things are done" in the culture of academic medicine.

As tempting as it may be to skip the step of genuinely understanding our CAS, some issues, in particular racism and bias, are too important to simply rely on the same approaches that have failed us in the past. We are capable of addressing pressing needs and managing crises, while also taking the time to think deeply, reflect, embrace uncertainty, and see every breakdown as a potential breakthrough.[7]

Taking an adaptive or living systems approach challenges many of our notions of how to think about causal relationships and how to make change. Making change in a living system requires understanding the context in which the problem occurs and demands both creativity and resourcefulness.

CREATIVE THINKING

Lewis Thomas, an American physician, poet, and essayist, observed, "When you are confronted by any complex social system … with things about it that you're dissatisfied with and anxious to fix, you cannot just step in and set about fixing with much hope of helping. This is one of the sore discouragements of our time." He went on to say, "If you want to fix something you are first obligated to understand . . . the whole system."[9]

Too often we treat the symptoms of systemic oppression in our CAS with a quick fix: a training, a policy, or some other action that does not address the underlying causes. Examples of these well-intentioned but ultimately inadequate fixes include increasing admissions diversity numbers, or explicitly naming racism in the MD curriculum. Once done, we check that box and move on to the next issue or problem to solve. This approach is transactional and relies on the completion of tasks to achieve a perceived goal or end result. Admittedly, the allure of concrete, short-term solutions, especially when they are relatively easy to achieve, is strong.

Adopting these solutions is often necessary but never sufficient for the task of CAS change. Moreover, this approach is deeply embedded in the very foundation and culture of academic medical institutions. Traditionally, physician leaders have depended on reasoning and logical, or "vertical," thinking to solve organizational problems.[10] This thinking is linear and employs a sequential method of solving problems, in which only one solution is generally realized. In many situations this style of thinking benefits us, especially if we need to deliver accurate information succinctly and quickly. Much of the instruction in undergraduate and graduate medical education focuses on developing this type of thinking. It is believed that this thinking "... produces physicians who are capable of making correct decisions under ambiguous circumstances, leading to the rigorous development of analytical, sequential thought processes that enable literature-supported, evidence-based decisions."[10] Although it might serve well in a clinical or research context, this type of thinking is not suited to address complex, chronic social problems such as racism. Vertical thinking oversimplifies the problems we are trying to solve, and all too often worsens and perpetuates them by providing a dangerously false sense of accomplishment and resolution.

If we want to address racism we need to think differently. This does not mean that we should completely abandon vertical thinking and swing the pendulum too far in the other direction. We need to learn to do both—indeed often simultaneously—so as to adapt our thinking and ultimately our actions, and avoid the default of solely relying on traditional ways of approaching problems.

In the next two sections of this chapter we highlight two important types of creative thinking: lateral or horizontal thinking, and systems thinking. At a high level, lateral thinking was developed as an alternative to step-by-step linear, or vertical thinking to generate new, out-of-the box ideas and solutions. Systems thinking has its origins in lateral thinking and can be described as the ability to see how things are interrelated and form a larger "whole." These two types of thinking are more aligned with transformational change in CASs.

Lateral or Horizontal Thinking

Lateral or horizontal thinking—a term first coined by physician and commentator Edward de Bono in 1967—allows us to identify different approaches to solving problems.[11] It is not sequential, linear, or necessarily logical, and it does not require us to determine the "right" answer. Instead, lateral or horizontal thinking demands that we gain a breadth of knowledge and acquire the skills to understand complex social systems. To do this we are called upon to reframe and question the root causes of the problems that we are trying to solve, search for alternatives that go beyond the obvious solutions, and expose ourselves to other disciplines that are more oriented towards lateral thinking. To illustrate the difference between linear or vertical thinking and lateral or horizontal thinking, imagine that you sit on the board of a nonprofit that is struggling financially. Vertical thinking may lead the board to suggest cost-cutting measures. Lateral thinking may lead the board to come up with creative new ways of partnering with another nonprofit that has shared goals and values.

For many of us, especially physicians, the uncertainty of novel and unconventional horizontal approaches can be unsettling, especially when there are abiding cultural and emotional pressures to find the "right" answer and to succeed all of the time. How to move beyond our discomfort and employ new ways of thinking is a challenge, but one we must undertake if we are to identify and address racism and other interlocking systems of oppression.

Systems Thinking

Systems thinking is based on systems theory and is responsible for one of the major breakthroughs in the understanding of complex organizations.[12] A mindset more than a prescribed practice, systems thinking investigates the connected wholes, rather than separate parts, that can contribute to a possible outcome.

Systems thinking differs from linear or vertical thinking in multiple ways. Table 2.1 provides a comparison.[13,14] The objective is to distinguish when it is beneficial to employ each of these types of thinking, depending on the problem at hand.

Adopting systems thinking requires persistence, practice, curiosity, and risk-taking. Being the sole systems thinker in a linear or vertical thinking institution can be lonely, even scary. Based on our experience, the linear thinkers around you will initially either be confused or actively resist this approach to addressing problems. With time, after witnessing the benefits of systems thinking, you will start to see a shift in how people react to and approach solving problems. Of course, it is important to acknowledge that many people are already oriented towards systems thinking, sometimes without even knowing that what they are doing is labeled systems thinking.

CHANGE IN COMPLEX ADAPTIVE SYSTEMS

The Greek philosopher Heraclitus is quoted as saying "change is the only constant in life." Even though this might be true, it does not mean that we understand change, especially in our work and learning environments. After conducting an extensive search of "thought leadership" on change, Freedman and Ghini found three common assumptions that, if not well understood, determine whether or not change is ultimately successful.[15]

The first assumption about change is that it is linear. This should not come as a surprise. When we think of change as linear we plan for change to have start and end points. Once we have decided that the plan or project is complete, the change is deemed complete. This approach to change is called "ready, aim, fire."[15] Although standard practice in medical schools, this approach does not take into consideration that change is never predictable or controllable. It is impossible to have a start and end in CAS. We need a way to conceptualize change as a living process with built-in mechanisms for continuous course correction as new information is revealed.

The second assumption is that change is primarily a cognitive process. The notion is that once individuals understand that the change is better for the institution or for themselves they will change. The mental model driving this belief is that a clear, logical case will promote change. This approach might work if

TABLE 2.1 Comparison Between Linear and Systems Thinking	
Linear (Vertical) Thinking	**Systems Thinking**
Institutions are predictable and orderly.	Institutions are unpredictable and are often a chaotic environment.
Connection between problems and their causes is obvious and easy to trace.	Relationships between problems and their causes are indirect and not obvious.
A policy designed to achieve short-term success will also assure long-term success.	Most quick fixes have unintended consequences. They may make no difference or make matters worse in the long run.
Break things into components or pieces.	Concerned with the whole, not just the parts.
Try to fix symptoms or react to events.	Concerned with underlying dynamics (structures, mental models, institutional and cultural values).
Concerned with assigning blame. Others, either within or outside our institution, are to blame for our problems and must be the ones to change.	Concerned with identifying patterns in the system. We unwittingly create our own problems and have significant control or influence in solving them through changing our patterns of behavior.
Try to control chaos to create order.	Try to find patterns amidst the chaos.
Concerned with content ("the what" – product, action, event, etc.).	Concerned with process ("the how" – engaging people, collaboration, feedback loops, course correction, etc.).
Aggressively tackle many independent initiatives simultaneously.	Only a few key coordinated changes sustained over time will produce large systems change.

humans were rational beings, but we are not, especially when confronted with change. While change is a normal part of our lives, it is uncomfortable for the vast majority of us because it makes us feel like we have lost control.

Change is never a neutral word. We cannot expect people to leave their emotions at the door when faced with change. In fact, we must consider the emotional impact and dynamics throughout the change process. In Fig. 2.1, the Change Curve is a model used to identify various emotional responses to change. Whatever the cause of the change, most people react in roughly the same way. They progress through a series of emotional stages, and do so at different paces. In addition, the curve is rarely linear. Individuals may cycle through the different emotional responses depending on the scale and type of change, what is happening in the CAS and in their personal lives.

The third assumption is that organizational change is driven by changing systems. Change efforts and strategic plans are often designed at the structural level but break down at the human level. Culture typically "eats strategy for breakfast."[18] Our strategies will not work if people will not or cannot execute them. Thus it is critical to place people at the center of the planning. That is why it is important to consider change management, or "… the application of a structured process and set of tools for leading the 'people side' of change to achieve a desired outcome."[19,20] Later in this chapter we provide additional information about change management.

Types of Change

Not all change is the same. What is the "right" type of change to effectively address racism and bias in a CAS? There are three different strata of change to consider (Fig. 2.2):

- Traditional or developmental change: focuses on making improvements to current practices while effectively maintaining the status quo.
- Transitional change: aims to change current practices to improve outcomes, with tangential impact on the status quo.
- Transformational change: aims to change not only practices, but the way in which we perceive, anticipate, and value outcomes, thereby disrupting the status quo.

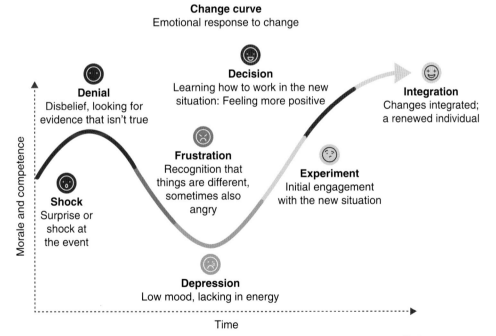

Fig. 2.1 Change Curve Model. (Adapted from Dr. Elisabeth Kubler-Ross Publication, 1969[16]; *FarWell*. Emotionally support employees during change: use the change curve as a conversation canvas. <https://gofarwell.com/how-leaders-can-emotionally-support-employees-during-change-use-the-change-curve-as-a-conversation-canvas/>[17]; Accessed 06.01.23.)

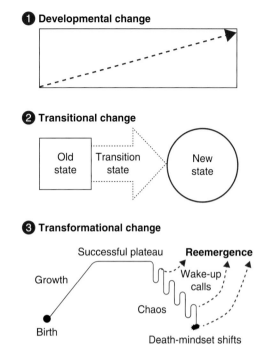

Fig. 2.2 Types of Change (From Anderson D, Anderson AA. What is transformation, and why is it so hard to manage? *Breakthrough Blog.* 2020.)

Developmental change improves previously established processes or procedures. There is a fixed problem to solve, a clear solution, and a finite desired outcome. For example, a medical school has an outdated learning management system, identifies a better alternative, purchases and implements it.

Transitional change is also linear but more broadly impactful, moving an organization from an "old" state to a "new," clearly defined state. For example, a hospital decides to become a health system by acquiring or merging with other local hospitals. A new organization is created, often imposing the policies, processes, and culture of the major hospital onto its smaller health system partners, while paying lip service to genuinely changing its culture.

Transformational change radically and fundamentally alters a culture, with an end result that is by definition unknown, and therefore daunting and unsettling. This change takes an institution from a steady state or plateau, through a series of chaotic episodes from which it reemerges ("wake-up calls"), until ultimately its previous mindset "dies" and an ever-evolving mindset is created.

For example, the future state of being an antiracist school of medicine cannot be known because it is radically different from the current state and there are no existing models. Through trial and error, as information comes in via feedback loops, the institution continuously becomes antiracist. This process is unpredictable, disruptive, and emergent; opportunities arise to transform breakdowns into breakthroughs. The difficulty here is compounded by the recognition that each CAS exists in a universe of interacting systems.

TRANSFORMATIONAL CHANGE PROCESS DYNAMICS

Transformation occurs through an intricate and complex process. There are four process dynamics of transformational change that are important to recognize before embarking on the journey.

First, transformational change is not easily managed. One needs to let go of the urge to control the change process rigidly, while still embracing the need for a navigation system or roadmap. In the next section we will present the antiracism change process roadmap to illustrate what we mean. One also has to be mindful that the system must continue to deliver regular results while this transformation is advancing.

Second, the process and outcomes of transformational change are emergent. Table 2.2 compares the difference between planned and emergent approaches to change.[20-22] There is a vast difference between being able to plan change and predict what will happen, and having faith that change will emerge over time with unforeseen circumstances and consequences. With emergent change, there will be setbacks and breakthroughs that one can learn to anticipate so that they do not derail the transformation.

Third, transformation requires a fullstream process that includes upstream, midstream, and downstream components.[23] Upstream intentionally sets the stage for the conditions of successful change; midstream focuses on designing the desired state; and downstream attends to implementation. All three components need to be consciously designed and facilitated for change to succeed in CASs. Fig. 2.3 illustrates the Fullstream Transformation Model.

Fourth, the process of planning, designing, and implementing the change must consider the content and people. In this case, content is what needs to change. We

TABLE 2.2 Planned Versus Emergent Approach to Change

Planned Change	Emergent Change
Controllable	Unpredictable and messy
Follows the intended strategy	Responds to events as they arise (e.g., changes in external environment)
Driven by management (top down)	Multilevel and cross-organizational
There is a clear beginning, middle, and end	Continual process of experimentation and adaptation with unforeseen events, disruptions, breakdowns, and opportunities that emerge
Assumption that there is full understanding of the consequences of actions, and that the plan will be understood, accepted, and be implemented fully	Believes in natural emergence of many factors during the change implementation phase that have never been forecast
Often ignores the realities of organizational conflict and politics	Acknowledges the developing and unpredictable nature of change in organizations

From Garcia-Lorenzo L, Liebhart M. Between planned and emergent change: decision maker's perceptions of managing change in organisations. *Int J Knowl Cult Change Manage Annu Rev.* 2010;10(5):147-162. doi:10.18848/1447-9524/cgp/v10i05/49976.

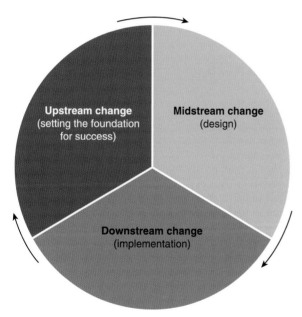

Fig. 2.3 Fullstream Transformation Model (From Anderson LA, Anderson D. *The Change Leader's Roadmap: How to Navigate Your Organization's Transformation.* Vol. 384. Hoboken, NJ: John Wiley & Sons; 2010.)

often focus on the "what" (content) and do not devote adequate time to the "how" (process) of getting there. In terms of people, we must consider how people change and we must be equipped to handle the human dynamics of change: people's mindsets, commitment, emotional reactions, behaviors, resistance, relationships,

politics, and cultural dynamics. For example, in changing a component of the curriculum it is clear what content needs to change. But are we focusing enough attention on the new way faculty will need to teach, the novel assessment methods that will be required, the impact on interdependent parts of the curriculum, the added burden to staff who have to support this change, and the emotional toll on all our constituents whenever we undertake such a change? In the next section of this chapter, we present an antiracist change process roadmap that is designed to incorporate all four process dynamics with creative thinking activities and antiracist practices.

ANTIRACIST CHANGE PROCESS ROADMAP

Drawing on the work of transformational change and change management leaders Anderson and Anderson,[7] and Kotter,[24] we designed a change process that includes five phases, each of which has a series of activities that include creative thinking approaches, tools, and antiracist practices. Fig. 2.4 illustrates the five phases.

Phase 1: Assessing Readiness for Change

During this phase, the focus is on assessing readiness for transformational change at the individual and school levels. This step begins to assess the existing landscape and the effectiveness of efforts that are already in place to address racism and bias.

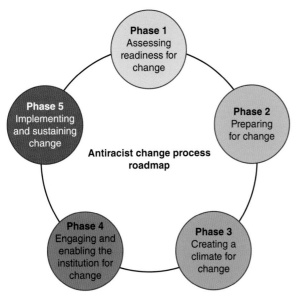

Fig. 2.4 Change Process Roadmap (Anderson LA, Anderson D. *The Change Leader's Roadmap: How to Navigate Your Organization's Transformation.* Vol. 384. Hoboken, NJ: John Wiley & Sons; 2010.)

Phase 2: Preparing for Change

During this phase, there is a focus on envisioning a future state of antiracist transformational change; identifying the elements and scope of change; and developing a change management strategy that includes identifying key roles, planning for resistance, and preparing leadership to sponsor the change.

Phase 3: Creating a Climate for Change

During this phase, there is an intentional focus on "being the change" by becoming deeply committed to the change process; continuing to practice and learn while eliciting feedback from those most affected by the change; building a powerful, enthusiastic group of change leaders (a Guiding Coalition) who will oversee the change strategy and process; and communicating the vision, strategy, and process for change across the institution.

Phase 4: Engaging and Enabling the Institution for Change

During this phase change targets (areas of focus), tactical plans, and frameworks for monitoring outcomes and performance are developed; the Guiding Coalition empowers broad-based action by building awareness, generating short-term wins, communicating clearly and

consistently with stakeholders, and creating opportunities to increase knowledge of key concepts related to racism and bias to support implementation of the change targets.

Phase 5: Implementing and Sustaining Change

During this phase there is a focus on embedding the change and ensuring that it sticks by actively pursuing information and feedback; learning from wins and mistakes; and turning that learning into appropriate course corrections. This process is not fixed or formulaic, but rather one that accelerates success by building the capacity to be agile and effectively operate within a state of uncertainty.

In the next five chapters we will introduce each phase in detail and provide instructions on how you can implement various change process roadmap activities in your own institution. We also provide many examples from our experience in implementing this antiracist roadmap at our school of medicine.[3]

REFERENCES

1. Kendi IX. *How to Be an Antiracist.* New York, NY: One World; 2015.
2. Cohen A, Rosenberg NO. Beehive or clockworks: complexity in execution. Insigniam; 2015. https://insigniam.com/wp-content/uploads/2020/11/Execution-Perspectives.pdf.
3. Hess L, Palermo AG, Muller D. Addressing and undoing racism and bias in the medical school learning and work environment. *Acad Med.* 2020;95(12S):S44-S50. doi:10.1097/acm.0000000000003706.
4. Joseph OR, Flint SW, Raymond-Williams R, Awadzi R, Johnson J. Understanding healthcare students' experiences of racial bias: a narrative review of the role of implicit bias and potential interventions in educational settings. *Int J Environ Res Public Health.* 2021;18(23):12771.
5. Redford G. *AAMC releases framework to address and eliminate racism.* AAMC. October 6, 2020. https://www.aamc.org/news/aamc-releases-framework-address-and-eliminate-racism.
6. Dooley KJ. A complex adaptive systems model of organization change. *Nonlinear Dynamics Psychol Life Sci.* 1997;1:69-97. https://doi.org/10.1023/A:1022375910940.
7. Anderson LA, Anderson D. *The Change Leader's Roadmap: How to Navigate Your Organization's Transformation.* Vol. 384. Hoboken, NJ: John Wiley & Sons; 2010.
8. Interaction Institute for Social Change. *Facilitative Leadership for Social Change.* https://interactioninstitute.org/training/facilitative-leadership-for-social-change-virtual/.

9. Stroh DP. *Systems Thinking for Social Change: A Practical Guide to Solving Complex Problems, Avoiding Unintended Consequences, and Achieving Lasting Results.* White River Junction, VT: Chelsea Green Publishing; 2015.

10. Hernandez JS, Varkey P. Vertical versus lateral thinking. *Physician Exec.* 2008;34(3):26-28.

11. Bono DE. *New Think: The Use of Lateral Thinking in the Generation of New Ideas.* New York, NY: Basic Books; 1967.

12. Stroh DP. *Systems Thinking for Social Change: A Practical Guide to Solving Complex Problems, Avoiding Unintended Consequences, and Achieving Lasting Results.* New York, NY: Chelsea Green Publishing; 2015.

13. Ollhaff J, Walcheski M. Making the jump to systems thinking - the systems thinker. The Systems Thinker. https://thesystemsthinker.com/making-the-jump-to-systems-thinking.

14. Acaroglu L. Disruptive Design: A Method for Activating Positive Social Change by Design. https://www.unschools.co/journal-blog/2020/2/22/week-41-sneak-peek-at-the-new-design-systems-change-handbook-by-leyla-acaroglu.

15. Freedman J, Ghini M. *Inside Change: Transforming Your Organization with Emotional Intelligence.* San Francisco, CA: Six Seconds Emotional Intelligence Press; 2010.

16. Kübler-Ross E. *On Death and Dying ; Questions and Answers on Death and Dying ; on Life after Death.* New York: Quality Paperback Book Club; 2002.

17. FarWell. How leaders can emotionally support employees during change: use the change curve as a conversation canvas. https://gofarwell.com/how-leaders-can-emotionally-support-employees-during-change-use-the-change-curve-as-a-conversation-canvas/.

18. Board TA. *"Culture Eats Strategy for Breakfast" - What Does It Mean?* https://www.thealternativeboard.com/blog/culture-eats-strategy#:~:text=The%20culture%20eats%20strategy%20for,that%20make%20all%20the%20difference

19. Hiatt J. *ADKAR: A Model for Change in Business, Government and our Community.* Loveland, CO: Prosci Research; 2006.

20. Prosci Inc. *The Global Leader in Change Management Solutions.* https://www.prosci.com/?utm_term=prosci&utm_campaign=ADKAR&utm_source=adwords&utm_medium=ppc&hsa_acc=5529787200&hsa_cam=10286811822&hsa_grp=114407014760&hsa_ad=474863235037&hsa_src=g&hsa_tgt=kwd-149880997&hsa_kw=prosci&hsa_mt=p&hsa_net=adwords&hsa_ver=3&gclid=CjwKCAiAh9qdBhAOEiwAvxIokyjv1jIPaDNqSgYBYXKEcH9KOTuMpFrC28HV9AmJFlIR1b-xJBpUCRoCu0MQAvD_BwE.

21. Anderson D, Anderson AA. What is transformation, and why is it so hard to manage? Breakthrough Blog. https://blog.beingfirst.com/what-is-transformation-and-why-is-it-so-hard-to-manage.

22. Spacey J. *Change: Emergent vs Planned.* Simplicable. https://simplicable.com/new/emergent-change.

23. Garcia-Lorenzo L, Liebhart M. Between planned and emergent change: decision maker's perceptions of managing change in organisations. *Int J Knowl Cult Change Manag Annu Rev.* 2010;10(5):147-162. doi:10.18848/1447-9524/cgp/v10i05/49976.

24. Kotter JP. *Leading Change: An Action Plan from the World's Foremost Expert on Business Leadership.* Boston, MA: Harvard Business Review Press; 2012.

Phase 1: Assessing Readiness for Change

CHAPTER OUTLINE

Readiness for Change
Antiracist Practice: Critical Self-Reflection
Three Assessments to Determine Readiness for Change

Phase 1 Activities and Instructions
   Activity 1a: Personal Change-Readiness Assessment
   Activity 1b: Sponsor Readiness Assessment
   Activity 1c: Organizational Change-Readiness Assessment

Antiracist Change Process Roadmap: Phase 1:

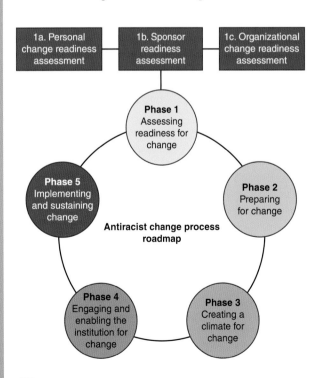

READINESS FOR CHANGE

Institutions do not change, people do.

It is the people within an institution who must shift from the current state to the desired future state, including the process of transitioning between those two states. Ideally, when taking on a transformational change such as antiracism we want people to be ready, exert effort, persevere in the face of obstacles, display cooperative behavior, and align with the vision.

Change management experts have long emphasized the importance of establishing organizational readiness for change. Change readiness is "a shared psychological state in which organizational members feel committed to implementing an organizational change and confident in their abilities to do so. Individuals must be both willing and able to put new mindsets and practices in place for change to happen."[2] Conceptually it makes sense that before implementing change it is important to determine if the institution is ready for it. In practice, this step is often skipped, and is not as straightforward as it seems. What does it mean to be "ready" or to assess readiness? What does it mean to achieve readiness for antiracist change? To make the journey easier for those involved, it is imperative to first assess and recognize organizational change readiness.

As Weiner[2] describes, organizational change readiness is a multilevel and multifaceted construct. For example, readiness can be present at the individual, group, unit, department, or organizational levels.[2] It has two conceptually interrelated facets—change commitment and change efficacy—that focus on cognitive and motivational aspects of readiness. Weiner goes on to suggest that change commitment is a function of change valence. Simply put, do people value the specific impending change? Do they think it is needed, important, beneficial, and worthwhile?

Change efficacy, on the other hand, is the "cognitive appraisal of three determinants of implementation capability: task demands, resources available, and situational factors.[2]" For example, what effort will it take to implement this change effectively? Do we have the resources to implement this change effectively? Can we implement this change effectively given the situation we currently face? Thus implementation capability is contingent upon identifying and understanding the determinants of organization readiness for change, as outlined in Fig. 3.1.

This chapter invites those planning for antiracist transformational change to identify their personal change readiness based on common traits; explore leadership change readiness as it relates to their change sponsorship role; and identify the determinants of readiness for organizational change. The chapter also provides the assessment tools to accomplish that. To the best of our knowledge there is no known validated tool to assess readiness for change as it relates to antiracism. Thus we have adapted various tools from available change management and antiracist organizational change assessment tools. We start by asking those embarking on this journey to employ the antiracist practice of critical self-reflection. In the following section, we provide a framework and Self-Reflection Questions for your consideration.

ANTIRACIST PRACTICE: CRITICAL SELF-REFLECTION

Critical self-reflection requires engaging in a process of analyzing and making judgments about one's experiences.[3,4] This process is understood as a "conscious exploration" or "deep deliberate search" where we observe, ask questions, identify patterns, and put facts, ideas, and experiences together to derive new meaning and self-understanding. Self-reflection is a necessary step towards becoming antiracist. It allows you to gain insight into your own beliefs and socialization, and uncover how you relate to others and larger systems.

Using the framework[5] outline that follows, we recommend taking the time to self-reflect prior to embarking on your change process journey.[5]

- *Reflecting on self.* Pose racially and culturally grounded questions about yourself to increase your awareness of seen (known), unseen (unknown), and unforeseen (unanticipated) issues.
- *Reflecting on self in relation to others.* Acknowledge the multiple roles, identities, and positions you and others bring to the change process.
- *Shifting from self to system.* Consider how history, politics, and your institution's culture share your racialized ways of being in your work and learning environments.

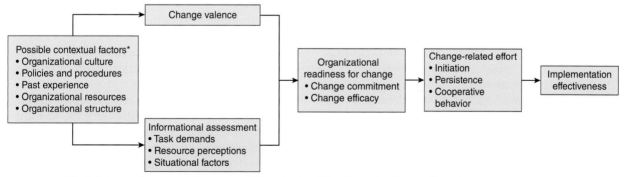

Fig. 3.1 Determinants and Outcomes of Organizational Readiness for Change (From Weiner BJ. A theory of organizational readiness for change. *Implement Sci.* 2009;4(67). doi:10.1186/1748-5908-4-67.)[2]

Potential Self-Reflection Questions:

- *Reflecting on self:*
  - What is my racial and/or cultural heritage? How do I know?
  - In what ways do my racial and cultural backgrounds influence how I experience the world, what I emphasize in my role, and how I evaluate and interpret others and their experiences? How do I know?
  - What do I believe about race and culture in society, medical education, and academic medicine, and how do I attend to my own convictions and beliefs about race and culture in my role?
  - What have been the contextual nuances and realities that helped shape my racial and cultural way of knowing, both past and present?
- *Reflecting on self in relation to others:*
  - What is the racial and/or cultural heritage of those with whom I work or learn? How do I know?
  - In what ways do my colleagues'/classmates' racial and cultural backgrounds influence how they experience the world? How do I know?
  - What do my colleagues/classmates believe about race and culture in society and medical education? How do they and I attend to the tensions inherent in those beliefs? How do I know?
  - What have been the contextual nuances and realities that have shaped my colleagues'/classmates' racial and cultural ways of knowing, both past and present? How consistent are their realities with mine? How do I know?
- *Shifting from self to system:*
  - What is the contextual nature of race, racism, and culture in my school and the broader community? How do I know?
  - What is known socially, institutionally, and historically about medical school and the broader community?
  - What do marginalized racial and cultural groups say about medical school and the broader community?
  - What systemic and organizational barriers and structures shape peoples' experiences in medical school and in the broader community?

Even though this is a personal practice, we invite you to debrief as a group. Consider the themes, differences, and similarities that were generated. Are there any insights that should be considered at this time? Any next steps that you should be taking?

THREE ASSESSMENTS TO DETERMINE READINESS FOR CHANGE

The three assessments outlined in this section will help those who are planning antiracist transformational change to determine readiness for change on personal, leadership (sponsor), and institutional levels. The intention is to use these self-assessment tools to further understand the landscape in which the change will occur and help inform the design of the upcoming change process phases. Conducting these assessments is not meant to be formal research or provide statistical findings.

PHASE 1 ACTIVITIES AND INSTRUCTIONS

Activity 1a: Personal Change-Readiness Assessment

We all experience and deal with change in different ways. It is important to understand oneself. What are your main strengths and obstacles when it comes to dealing with change? The Purdue Change-Readiness Assessment includes statement questions and focuses on the seven traits of personal change readiness: resourcefulness, optimism, adventurousness, passion/drive, adaptability, confidence, and tolerance for ambiguity.[6] Please note that the questionnaire is designed for self-reflection and personal development only. It is not intended to measure performance or capability when faced with change.

Time expected to complete: 30 minutes.

Target audience: Those involved in planning the change.

Purpose of the activity: To assess the seven traits related to your own change readiness.

Instructions:

- Access the Purdue Change-Readiness Assessment[6]: https://www.ecfvp.org/files/uploads/2_-change_readiness_assessment_0426111.pdf?trk=article-ssr-frontend-pulse_little-text-block and answer the 35 questions.
- Add the scores for the questions in each of the trait categories. Understand your score by reading the seven trait descriptions.
- Debrief with others who are involved in planning the change. This could include discussing the strengths and opportunities related to your personal change readiness traits and determining which roles might be a good fit for you. For example, adventurers are great starters, resourceful people are excellent problem solvers, optimists make good cheerleaders and their input is especially useful when people feel discouraged.

Activity 1b: Sponsor Readiness Assessment

According to Prosci's two decades of best practices in change management research,[7] executive sponsors have a critical role to play during times of change.[7] An executive sponsor is a leader who authorizes the change and is ultimately responsible for ensuring that the change realizes its intended benefits (see Chapter 4 for a detailed role description). Based on Prosci's research, we have adapted questions that can be used to assess if the sponsor is aware and able to use best practices to promote change.[7] Information gathered from this tool can be used to help coach the sponsor throughout the process.

Time expected to complete: 1 hour.

Target audience: Those involved in planning the change.

Purpose of the activity: To assess sponsor readiness to change.

Instructions:
- Schedule a meeting with those involved in planning the change.
- Enabling sponsors involves preparing, equipping, and supporting the appropriate leader to fulfill their critical responsibilities. As a group, review the definition provided below and the *ABCs of sponsorship roles*, and identify who the sponsors are within your medical school or institution.
  - *Definition.* Executive and senior leaders play an essential role as primary sponsors of change. They give the change credibility, authorize funding and resources, and perform important employee-facing activities. People in the institution look to these individuals at the top to demonstrate why the change is necessary and to perform other critical activities as only they can.
  - There are three actions or behaviors associated with the success of the sponsor role. These are called the ABCs of sponsorship:
    - *Active* and visible participation throughout the project
    - *Build* a team of support
    - *Communicate* directly with constituents about the reasons for and nature of the change
- As a group, answer the Sponsor Readiness Questions that follow. Be sure to document answers in Worksheet 3.1.

Sponsor Readiness Questions

Are your sponsors:
- aware of their importance in making change successful?
- aware of their biggest roles in supporting the project?
- active and visible throughout the change initiative?
- building the coalition necessary for change to be successful?
- communicating directly and effectively with people who will be impacted?
- aware that the biggest mistake is failing to personally engage as the sponsor?
- prepared to manage resistance?
- prepared to celebrate successes?
- setting and reconciling clear priorities regarding this change, other initiatives, and day-to-day work?
- avoiding the "flavor of the month" syndrome?

As a group, reflect on the following:
- What are your initial thoughts/reactions to the answers?
- What are the answers that surprised you and should be reexamined? Why? Is there something not being said?
- What are the next steps in selecting sponsors (if not already selected) and getting them ready?
- How will sponsors engage throughout the life of the change process?

Activity 1c: Organizational Change-Readiness Assessment

Since there is no single assessment tool that includes readiness to change (as outlined earlier) and the conditions that can signal where the institution is in relation to antiracism readiness, we have identified questions from multiple tools. Here you will find examples of questions adapted from a validated Readiness Scale,[8] Transforming Organizational Capacity Assessment[9] (TOCA), and the Washington Race Equity & Justice Initiative (REJI) Organizational Assessment.[10]

Readiness Scale information assessment[8] (1 = "strongly disagree," 5 = "strongly agree," unsure):
1. People who work or learn here believe we have the expertise we need to implement this change.
2. People who work or learn here believe we have the time we need to implement this change.
3. People who work or learn here believe we have the skills we need to implement this change.
4. People who work or learn here believe we have the resources we need to implement this change.
5. People who work or learn here know how much time it will take to implement this change.
6. People who work or learn here know what resources we will need to implement this change.

7. People who work or learn here know what each of us has to do to implement this change.

Change commitment and change efficacy:

8. People who work or learn here are committed to implementing this change.
9. People who work or learn here are determined to implement this change.
10. People who work or learn here are motivated to implement this change.
11. People who work or learn here will do whatever it takes to implement this change.
12. People who work or learn here want to implement this change.
13. People who work or learn here feel confident they can keep the momentum going in implementing this change.
14. People who work or learn here feel confident they can manage the politics of implementing this change.
15. People who work or learn here feel confident the organization can support people as they adjust to this change.
16. People who work or learn here feel confident that the organization can get people invested in implementing this change.
17. People who work or learn here feel confident they can coordinate tasks so that implementation goes smoothly.
18. People who work or learn here feel confident that they can track the progress in implementing this change.
19. People who work or learn here feel confident they can handle the challenges that might arise in implementing this change.

Transforming Organizational Capacity Assessment[9] (TOCA) (1= "strongly disagree," 5 = "strongly agree," unsure)

1. Most of our leaders support people who openly share situations involving racism and/or racial microaggressions in our medical school.
2. If someone raises an issue about racism, typically the person is marginalized and/or receives pushback for raising the issue.
3. Most of our staff have the confidence and skills to give feedback about situations involving race or racism.
4. Most of our leadership lacks the confidence and skills to give feedback about situations involving race or racism.

5. Giving feedback to our staff members about a comment made or attitude expressed about race/racism is typically not welcomed.
6. Giving feedback to our leadership about a comment made or attitude expressed about racism is typically welcomed.
7. Discussing whether or how a decision may be reinforcing white dominant culture and/or privileging whiteness in our medical school is encouraged by leadership.
8. Discussing the impact of a decision and whether racial inequities may result (even unintentionally) is not welcomed by our leadership.
9. Our policies are applied consistently, equitably, and transparently.
10. People with the most relevant lived experiences and/or who are most impacted by the decision are able to provide input into policymaking.
11. Our leaders prioritize their accountability to the Trustees, accrediting bodies, and/or donors, rather than to the people most impacted by their decisions.
12. Power to make decisions and communicate them is generally held by a select few with positional power in our medical school, and decisions are typically shared on an as-needed basis.
13. Only numbers and hard data are prioritized in assessing progress.
14. A diverse group (identity and positional power) define what progress and success look like at our institution.
15. Time is typically a major barrier to working on diversity, inclusion, and/or equity outcomes.
16. Racial equity goals are part of our strategic plan and each faculty and employee's performance evaluation.
17. The group designated to manage the diversity, equity, and inclusion (D/E/I) work in our medical school is limited in their power and resources to ensure D/E/I goals are met.

Race Equity & Justice Initiative[10] (REJI) organizational assessment (1= "strongly disagree," 5 = "strongly agree," unsure):

1. Our medical school creates space for discussing issues of race and racism in ways that are relevant to our work.
2. Cultural norms of our medical school, spoken or unspoken, allow for questions, issues, and concerns

about racial dynamics to be openly discussed and addressed.

3. Team members cannot meaningfully engage and work through tension when conflict arises.

4. Staff/leadership/volunteers/students who identify as people of color or as belonging to other historically marginalized groups can bring their full identities to our workplace and learning environment if they choose to and feel recognized and respected.

5. Staff who identify as people of color or as belonging to other historically marginalized groups can contribute to shaping our medical school culture.

6. Patients and community members feel welcome and comfortable entering our environment without having to conform to dominant (White) cultural expectations.

7. Our medical school does not encourage ideas, strategies, initiatives, and feedback from all stakeholders (including frontline staff, volunteers, patients, students), only those with positional authority.

8. When planning internal meetings and gatherings, our medical school considers accessibility and inclusion factors like language access/interpretation, accommodations, childcare, food, and location.

9. People are not aware of the forces driving change that exist outside our medical school.

10. Our medical school has successfully implemented change initiatives in the past.

11. The reason or the "why" of the coming change cannot easily be translated into tangible evidence that will get the attention of our students, faculty, and staff.

12. Our students, faculty, and staff feel a sense of urgency for change.

Time expected to complete: 30 min.

Target audience: This survey can be sent to anyone who can inform organizational change readiness.

Purpose of the activity: To assess organizational change readiness.

Instructions:

- Create a survey using the questions outlined earlier or other questions that can inform organizational change readiness.
- Once the data is analyzed, we recommend facilitating a meeting with those planning the change to review the data as it reflects your landscape before

moving on to the next phase: preparing for change. Use these questions to guide the discussion:

- What are three words/short phrases you would use to describe your medical school's culture?
- What are your medical school's current strengths and skills that will be helpful in creating an antiracist institution and culture? What strengths and skills do you bring in helping create a racially equitable medical school and culture?
- What are your medical school's challenges and/or barriers to creating an antiracist institution? What types of support are needed to address these challenges/barriers?

REFERENCES

1. Anderson LA, Anderson D. *The Change Leader's Roadmap: How to Navigate Your Organization's Transformation*. Vol. 384. Hoboken, NJ: John Wiley & Sons; 2010.
2. Weiner BJ. A theory of organizational readiness for change. *Implement Sci*. 2009;4(67). doi:10.1186/1748-5908-4-67.
3. Bart M. *Critical Reflection Adds Depth and Breadth to Student Learning*. Faculty Focus; 2017. http://www.facultyfocus.com/articles/instructional-design/critical-reflection-adds-depth-and-breadth-to-student-learning/.
4. Jacoby B. *How Can I Promote Deep Learning Through Critical Reflection?* Magna Publications; 2021. https://www.magnapubs.com/product/program/how-can-i-promote-deep-learning-through-critical-reflection/.
5. Milner R. Race, culture, and researcher positionality: working through dangers seen, unseen, and unforeseen. *Educ Res*. 2007;36(7):388-400.
6. ECF Vital Practices. *Change-Readiness Assessment*. https://www.ecfvp.org/files/uploads/2_-change_readiness_assessment_0426111.pdf.
7. Prosci. *Primary Sponsor's Role and Importance*. 2022. https://www.prosci.com/resources/articles/primary-sponsors-role-and-importance.
8. Shea CM, Jacobs SR, Esserman DA, Bruce K, Weiner BJ. Organizational readiness for implementing change: a psychometric assessment of a new measure. *Implement Sci*. 2014;9(7):1-15. doi:10.1186/1748-5908-9-7.
9. MP Associates. *Transforming Organizational Culture Assessment Tool (TOCA)*. 2020. http://www.mpassociates.us/uploads/3/7/1/0/37103967/toca_toolpotapchuk_.pdf.
10. JustLead Washington. *Reji Organizational Race Equity Toolkit*. 2nd ed. https://justleadwa.org/wp-content/uploads/2020/11/REJI-Toolkit-v2-Final-2020-3.pdf.

4

Phase 2: Preparing for Change

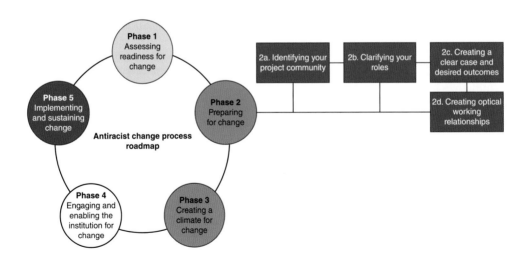

PLANTING THE SEEDS OF SUCCESSFUL TRANSFORMATION

As discussed in Chapter 2, the process of change requires full-stream transformation that includes upstream, midstream, and downstream components.[1] In this chapter, we will focus on *upstream* activities that will help you lay the foundation needed for successful antiracist change.

Most change efforts do not devote enough time upstream.[1] A sense of urgency to implement (to get to the "doing") takes over. We become focused on putting out fires and fixing problems. This type of urgency is even more heightened when we know that existing mindsets, practices, and structures produce ongoing inequity and harm. It makes sense to want to "fix" racism and identify solutions in our work and learning environments as fast as possible. The challenge is that a "fix" mindset often defaults to checking boxes and treating symptoms as markers of productivity and achievement. When we do that we are also more inclined to jump to a solution instead of valuing, and learning from, the process of getting there.

What would happen if we redefined what it means to do the work of antiracism well, or what it means to be productive? What if we considered the process of setting the conditions for success as "the work," as opposed to the busy work of completing tasks? What if we invested in the upstream, knowing that we will be more successful in the downstream, and ultimately lead to real change?

Drawing on the work of Anderson and Anderson, this chapter will outline four steps of preparing for change.[1] We will provide detailed instructions on how to execute each of the four steps (we call them "activities"), and where applicable we will share our experience as it relates to the change process. First, we invite those participating in the four steps of preparing for change to consider employing antiracist practices while completing the activities in this phase and the rest of the change process. In the next section, we have outlined details about how to begin to build or enhance a culture of accountability.

ANTIRACIST PRACTICE: ACCOUNTABILITY

The question of *accountability* often gets raised when talking about how to address racism in institutions. We have all heard things like, "We need to hold the leaders accountable." "We won't see real change unless it comes from the top." "It doesn't matter what we do. If we want to see change, we must have buy-in from the C-suite." When examining these statements it is clear they are influenced by hierarchical structures that rely solely on top-down management. This type of accountability is a command-and-control structure, which is a traditional organizational model where a single leader or group of leaders exerts complete control over all decision-making and communication within the organization.[2] When it comes to promoting change the assumption is that power and decision-making remain with those at the top. When it comes to addressing racism in a

complex adaptive system (CAS), a command-and-control structure with top-down management does not produce the results we want to see. For example, researchers have found that mandated training programs actually hurt diversity and can lead to what is called "backfire effect."[3] Some employees may feel threatened because of the loss of autonomy related to mandatory training. As a result, these employees ignore the training messaging, while some even go out of their way to defy it.

The unpredictable nature of CAS makes it problematic to implement traditional accountability, especially in systems that are self-organizing. Instead of being held accountable to outcomes or outputs, individuals and groups should be held accountable for learning, shared meaning making, directional movement, and individual and collective contributions to the culture. This type of accountability is more aligned with transformational change, especially when the future state or outcome is unknown and we cannot know what we will be holding ourselves accountable for as it relates to outcomes.

What if accountability is considered more of a practice? When it comes to addressing racism, we know that accountability is an integral part of addressing key characteristics within ourselves, in our relationships, and in our communities. Individuals, groups, and communities can intentionally work to build a culture of accountability.[4] The following text provides details about the three types of accountability that can be integrated throughout this phase and the entire antiracist change process.

Self-accountability is the practice of taking responsibility for your actions and the consequences of those actions. As a practice, individuals can engage in self-reflection to examine their own behaviors and develop their capacity to take responsibility. Here are some self-reflection questions that we have adapted for your consideration.[5]

Self-Reflection Questions:

- How often do you say or do something (e.g., make a comment, ask a question, or behave/react in a way) that is rooted in a racist attitude, assumption, or stereotype? (This includes things you think, say, or do in the presence of other people *and* things you think, say, or do that other people might not know about.)
- When you say or do something rooted in a racist attitude, assumption, or stereotype, what emotional

response does it bring up for you? (This includes the emotions you feel in the moment, whether in the presence of other people or alone, and the emotions you feel later on.)
- When you say or do something rooted in a racist attitude, assumption, or stereotype, what intellectual response does it bring up for you? Examples include but are not limited to rationalization (you lacked bad intent), awareness of the need for unlearning, acknowledgment of the impact on others, and recognizing your own internalized racism.
- When you say or do something rooted in a racist attitude, assumption, or stereotype in the presence of other people, how often do you acknowledge/name it to others without being called out for it first?
- When other people point out that you said or did something rooted in a racist attitude, assumption, or stereotype, what are your behavioral impulses? Do you explain your intent (what you did/did not mean), ask them to educate you, question their experience or interpretation, think or say they are overreacting, react to or comment on their tone, cause more harm with your comments/actions, verbally acknowledge accountability, apologize for the impact and harm?

Mutual accountability is the practice of using an explicit enforcement mechanism(s) that allows dyads and groups to hold those who have made commitments (or still need to make commitments) responsible for following through. Mutual accountability challenges group members to move beyond defensiveness, and commit to putting relationships ahead of the need to be right or be perceived as a "good person." Instead, the group focuses on the effects of the behavior and works to repair the harm caused. The Guiding Coalition and change strategy team (these roles are described in Activity 2b: Clarifying Your Roles) can use these discussion questions to uncover where they are at in terms of building mutual accountability.

Group discussion questions[6]:
- In what ways do we name harmful patterns and behaviors in the moment?
- Do we practice vulnerability and honesty about how we continue to learn and grow around racial equity and antiracism? If so, in what ways? If not, why do we think that is?

- To what extent are we open to feedback (1:1 or in a group) without getting defensive?
- To what extent do we take an active and engaged role in interrupting dominant cultural patterns and norms and prevent their replication?
- In what ways do we acknowledge that the systems that are failing communities of color are negatively affecting all of us, albeit in different ways?
- In what ways are we proactive about reaching out to those most affected (people of color), rather than waiting for them to come forward?
- To what extent do we strike a balance between speaking up, and stepping back to let others lead?

After discussing these questions, if there is a need to introduce and commit to an explicit mechanism that supports mutual accountability in naming and addressing harmful behaviors, we recommend using the ACTION model, as outlined in Fig. 4.1. The ACTION model is an inquiry-based tool to use during group interactions, whether in-person, virtual, or even in emails.[7]

Community accountability is the practice of creating communal support for those impacted and/or collectively interrupting, challenging, stopping, and shifting abusive behavior and the underlying systems that support it. This is an approach pioneered by feminists of color in the early 2000s. INCITE! Women of Color Against Violence defines it as a process in which a community works together to do the following[8]:
- Create and affirm values and practices that resist abuse and oppression and encourage safety, support, and accountability.
- Develop sustainable strategies to address community members' abusive behavior, creating a process for them to account for their actions and transform their behavior.
- Commit to ongoing development of all members of the community, and the community itself, to transform the political conditions that reinforce oppression and violence.
- Provide safety and support to community members who are violently targeted that respects their self-determination.

Throughout this process members of the Guiding Coalition are encouraged to explore how they will work with the project community (defined in the next section) to ensure accountability.

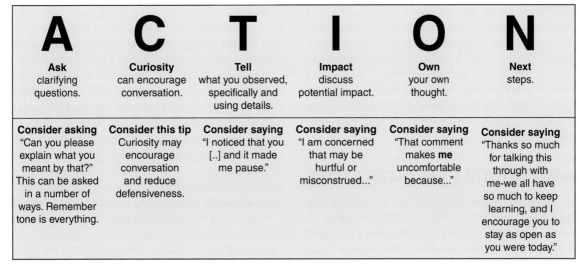

A Ask clarifying questions.	**C** Curiosity can encourage conversation.	**T** Tell what you observed, specifically and using details.	**I** Impact discuss potential impact.	**O** Own your own thought.	**N** Next steps.
Consider asking "Can you please explain what you meant by that?" This can be asked in a number of ways. Remember tone is everything.	**Consider this tip** Curiosity may encourage conversation and reduce defensiveness.	**Consider saying** "I noticed that you [..] and it made me pause."	**Consider saying** "I am concerned that may be hurtful or misconstrued..."	**Consider saying** "That comment makes **me** uncomfortable because..."	**Consider saying** "Thanks so much for talking this through with me-we all have so much to keep learning, and I encourage you to stay as open as you were today."

Fig. 4.1 ACTION Model (Souza T. *Responding to Microaggressions in the Classroom: Taking Action*. Faculty Focus; 2018. https://www.facultyfocus.com/articles/effective-classroom-management/responding-to-micro-aggressions-in-the-classroom/.)

FOUR STEPS OF PREPARING FOR CHANGE

These four steps do not need to be completed in order, although we have scaffolded these steps so that they build on one another. We recommend that you treat these steps as iterative and continue to update or refine them as new information becomes available. It is critically important to consider who needs to participate in the activities associated with each step, and the voices and perspectives that are often absent and need to be included.

Identifying Your Project Community

The first step is to identify and map out your project community so that you can clarify and specify whose realities the change effort is affecting and who needs to be involved in the process. At the start, we recommend that you identify and map everyone—internally and externally—who has a stake in the antiracist change and is engaged in or affected by it; this is your project community. This mapping will provide you with an easy reference for thinking through various stakeholder needs and the roles needed to shape your change strategy.

Clarifying Your Roles

The next step is to consider the various change roles needed to support your effort. For example, who will sponsor the effort, who will design and lead the change

strategy, and who will be involved in various other ways? Clear roles and responsibilities will minimize redundancy and ensure full coverage. These roles are a departure from more traditional task force or committee roles.

Creating a Clear Case and Desired Outcome

Now that you are clear about your project community and change roles, it is time to create a case for change and determine the initial desired outcomes that will inform and compel people to support and adopt the change. No one will invest their time and heart in the complex and challenging effort of transformation unless they understand why the change is necessary and what benefits it promises, personally and institutionally. This step answers the basic questions: "Why transform?" "What is at stake if we do not change?" "What needs to transform?" "What big picture outcomes do we want from this transformation?" and "What is included or not included in the scope of change?"

Creating Optimal Working Relationships

As a last step, it is imperative to intentionally focus on relationships to ensure the project community and those involved in planning and leading the change can sustain the work towards the desired outcome. It should come as no surprise that building and sustaining effective working relationships is an important condition for success. When people take on special change roles, it is essential to clarify the working relationships among them, and between them and their peers who retain existing functional roles. Too often, historical social and "political" tensions will surface as "toxins" and hinder you from accomplishing what the change effort requires. By addressing historical conflicts you can ensure the clearest thinking and behavior to support the overall transformation.

PHASE 2 ACTIVITIES AND INSTRUCTIONS

In the previous section we outlined four activities to help you prepare for change, including detailed instructions on how to complete each step. We have also provided suggestions for the target audience or who could participate in the activity, and the allotted time it might take to complete. These are suggested guidelines, and they should not impede your progress. We recommend that you determine what is needed and how much time it should take to complete the activities based on your institutional priorities. Resist the urge to just "check the box" when completing the activities. We invite you to treat these activities as a process: some will never be complete and might change as new information becomes available. We have also provided worksheets that can be used to document and share activity information with those involved in preparing for change.

Activity 2a: Identifying Your Project Community

The project community is a map of the individuals and groups that will be involved in the antiracism transformational change. As outlined by Anderson and Anderson,[1] a project community map should be able to answer the following questions: "Whose realties is the change effort affecting and who needs to be involved in some way?" "Who has a vested interest in the results?" "Who has something to offer, whether knowledge, skills, or resources?" "Who is going to be seriously impacted by the change?" and "Whose voices need to be heard?"

When identifying your project community, start by identifying everyone—internally and externally—who has a stake in the effort and is engaged in or affected by it. Consider various departments, functional areas, students, patients, faculty, staff, clerkship directors, etc. If your institution has individuals and groups already activated and engaged in antiracism work, you might want to start with them and build the map from there. Overall, this

identification will provide you an easy reference for thinking through various stakeholder needs as you shape your change strategy and develop your communications, resistance management plans, and sponsor roadmap.

The instructions that follow will help you facilitate the project community mapping. We recommend you schedule a meeting or a series of meetings with internal and external representatives who have a stake in the change and are engaged in or affected by it to complete the activity as a group. After the meeting, those planning next steps are encouraged to answer the postactivity self-reflection questions and follow up on any action items.

Time expected to complete activity: 1 hour meeting; might need to facilitate a series of meetings with different stakeholder groups.

Target audience: This activity will require you to meet with a group of people who can ensure your ultimate project community map is representative of everyone internally and externally who has a stake in the effort and is engaged in or affected by the antiracist change.

Purpose of the activity: To provide clarity and an easy reference for thinking through various stakeholder needs as you shape your change strategy and plans.

Instructions:
1. During the meeting:
   a. Ask the project community the questions listed in the Appendix, Worksheet 4.1.
   b. Record answers to the questions and fill out a grid in Activity 2a: Identifying Your Project Community (Worksheet 4.1).
2. After the meeting:
   a. Individually complete the Self-Reflection Questions.
   b. Create a mind map or other graphic representation of the project community.
   c. Follow up on any action items.

Project Community Mind Map

It will be easier to communicate the boundaries of the project community with a visual aid. Consider using a mind map to graphically organize the various stakeholders who will be involved in the transformational change effort. A mind map is a visual information management tool that helps to structure, organize, and arrange information in a specialized way.[9] There are online tools such as MindMeister or Mural that can be used to develop a mind map of your project community. You will find an example of a mind map in Fig 4.2.

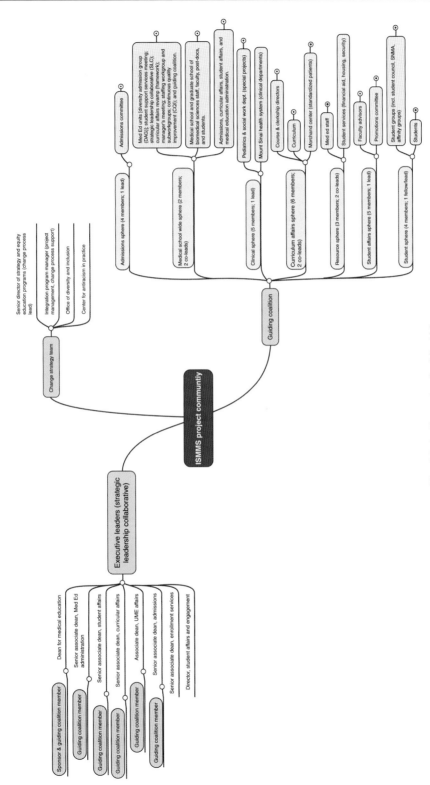

Fig. 4.2 An Example of a Mind Map.

Our Experience: Identifying the Project Community

This step took several months to complete because of our ongoing dialogue between department leadership and the Anti-Racism Coalition (ARC) student group (see Chapter 8 for more information about ARC). Initially, we went through several iterations of scoping out who should and who must be included in our project community. Each dialogue generated challenging, provocative, and deeply insightful discussions about where the problems lay in our complex work and learning environment. This step allowed us to deliberately step outside our silos in order to examine the MD program's systems and structures as a whole. We hoped to avoid focusing too narrowly and miscalculating the repercussions of the change we were envisioning. After much discussion among members of the medical education leadership team we decided that our project community would encompass the MD student learning environment from recruitment and admissions through the trajectory of the curriculum, the full scope of student affairs and diversity affairs, as well as student resources (financial aid, registrar, housing, etc.). While we unanimously agreed that taking on graduate medical education was beyond our capacity, there was significant debate about the clinical learning environment. On the one hand we had absolutely no influence over how care was practiced, structured, or compensated. On the other hand, the clinical environment was the crucible where our students would have their most valuable positive and negative learning experiences. In the end we chose to include a "clinical sphere" in an effort to account for that aspect of our students' learning environment.

Activity 2b: Clarifying Your Roles

The second step is to consider the various roles that are needed to achieve transformational change in a CAS. Anderson and Anderson note that taking on a change role is usually in addition to one's existing duties.[1] Therefore the various roles should be given to people who are the most competent and best positioned to successfully lead the effort. It is important to first consider which of the role responsibilities are already included in existing job functions and which responsibilities can be seamlessly integrated into existing roles.[1] This requires a great deal of open, honest conversation and even some vulnerability, as your change efforts will either be enhanced or encumbered by the role selections. When considering roles, we encourage you to have transparent conversations to minimize redundancy and ensure full

coverage of responsibilities. Make note and strategize if there are roles that cannot be fulfilled.

We have adapted the seven typical change roles for your consideration.[1] Read through each of these roles and proceed to the activity details.

Seven Typical Change Roles

Sponsor. Individual(s) with the highest line authority over the change effort based on the institutional hierarchical structure; executive champion; has primary influence over desired outcomes; actively and visibly participates throughout; builds networks by maintaining ongoing links with major stakeholders; communicates directly and delivers major communications; contributes to the change strategy; supports the change process leader; approves desired future state solutions; ensures conditions for success are named and supported; and models the desired mindset, behavior, and cultural changes required by the transformation.

Our Experience: Sponsor

As a free-standing medical school housed in a large academic health system, we have an organizational structure that presents opportunities and challenges when exercising high-impact decision-making authority and in securing sustained resources. Our organizational chart is flatter when compared to that of a medical school embedded in a university. At the same time, our health system's fiscal and programmatic priorities may influence the allocation of resources such as people, money, and space.

Our ARC students insisted that our Dean be present at the initial meeting they hosted in 2015, which subsequently catalyzed our journey to address racism and bias in medical education. The Dean expressed support for this initiative at the time and charged the Dean for Medical Education with this task, essentially appointing him to serve as the sponsor. This gave the Dean for Medical Education the opportunity to invite the Dean of the school to the very first all-student town hall, where the Racism and Bias Initiative (RBI) was introduced.

Since then it has been the Dean for Medical Education's responsibility to update the Dean regularly; include antiracism as a topic at all leadership meetings within medical education and among all deans and chairs; role model language, behaviors, and power-sharing that reflect our antiracism goals and objectives; and demonstrate lifelong learning.

Executive Team. Executive leadership team of the institution within which the change effort is occurring; responsible for desired outcomes in their designated functional areas; ensures priority of the overall change effort within the other priorities underway at the institution; models the desired mindset, behavior, and cultural changes required for success.

Our Experience: Executive Team

Our executive team includes the Dean for Medical Education, the respective senior associate and associate deans for admissions, student affairs, curricular affairs, diversity affairs, and medical education administration. We set an expectation that all executive team members join our Guiding Coalition and maintain an active presence in the RBI.

Because of lessons learned in our Guiding Coalition (see description below), we redesigned our executive team to reflect a far more diverse group of leaders and to provide a more strategic and equity-centered direction for the school. The redesigned leadership team included education leaders from additional areas, as well as some middle management staff, and became known as the Strategic Leadership Collaborative (SLC).

Change Strategy Team. Individuals with delegated authority to create and implement a multiphased antiracist change strategy (as outlined by the roadmap); ensures content, people, and process elements of the change are aligned; supports the Guiding Coalition as well as stakeholder groups and individuals towards the desired commitment for change that will be necessary to transform the project community; fosters understanding, acceptance. and ownership of the change within their functional area or sphere of influence; enables people to appreciate what they need to do differently to transform from the current state to the unknown future state; course-corrects along the way to constantly steer the strategy towards antiracism transformation; models the desired mindset, behavior, and cultural changes.

Our Experience: Change Strategy Team

Initially, this team was made up of select department staff who were interested in learning more about change management, and department leaders (executive team) who wanted to play a more hands-on role in designing the strategy. As time went on, the leaders became more focused on implementing the change in their respective spheres and staff stayed on because this became a valuable professional development opportunity.

We underestimated the importance of this change strategy team and what it could offer staff who often are not given professional development opportunities to build skills related to project management and change management.

Change Process Lead. A member of leadership or a manager who has delegated authority from the sponsor to lead the change effort and process; oversees design and execution of the change strategy and each phase of the change process; responsible for clarifying scope, desired outcomes, pace, conditions for success, constraints, and infrastructure; articulates the resources that will be needed for transformation; oversees communications and information management; ensures course correction; provides feedback and support to the change strategy team; models the desired mindset, behavior, and cultural changes.

Our Experience: Change Process Lead

The medical education leadership team was fortunate to have worked with Leona Hess, PhD, MSW on a consulting basis from 2016 to 2018, as described in Chapter 9. The team realized that we could not move forward with the change management process on our own. We needed specialized coaching and strategic guidance to articulate and achieve the vision. In 2018, the department of medical education and the office of diversity and inclusion worked with Dr. Hess to create the role of Senior Director of Equity and Strategy in Educational Programs, which positioned her as a member of the department of medical education's leadership team and provided joint salary support for this role. The joint financial investment and commitment between these two entities was a positive sign of progress towards partnership, and a shift away from a historically antagonistic relationship.

Guiding Coalition Members. Individuals from across the institution who contribute unique skills, experiences, perspectives, intersecting identities, and networks in order to enable the most innovative ideas to emerge; represent all areas of your project community; set direction for the change; oversee the change projects, actions, or initiatives (change targets); identify options and make decisions about where energy and resources should be focused; determine how to hold people accountable; manage resistance; muster support, buy-in, and resources from stakeholders and other parts of the institution and project community; model the desired mindset, behavior, and cultural changes.

Our Experience: Guiding Coalition Members

When determining who should be on the Guiding Coalition, we centered marginalized voices; ensured representation from all functional areas of the school; and considered positional power, social influence, expertise, credibility, and leadership ability. The work we did in defining our project community was helpful in framing who should participate, and in the organizational design of the Guiding Coalition. Since our focus was addressing racism and bias in the medical student learning environment, we needed to focus on all key functional areas of the medical school in the Guiding Coalition. Our design led to a model that included distinct spheres dedicated to students, admissions, curricular affairs, student affairs, student resources, and the clinical environment. In hindsight we came to realize that this model, while very effective, recreated and in some ways reinforced our existing silos. While this has not undermined our work, it has required us to be mindful of integration and bridging these spheres at every step of the way.

    Guiding Coalition Sphere Lead. An administrator or project manager who is in charge of overseeing planning with Guiding Coalition members so that results are achieved and people are engaged in positive ways; ensuring the change projects, actions or initiatives are being implemented and tracked within the Guiding Coalition sphere; may have their own supervisor, yet also reports to the change process lead; responsible for helping to set the change target(s) up for success; ensures timely course correction and coordination with interdependent and integrated change targets; models the desired mindset, behavior, and cultural changes.

Our Experience: Guiding Coalition Sphere Lead

Similar to the way we determined who should be on the Guiding Coalition, we were intentional about flattening the hierarchy so that the sphere leads did not have to be the most senior leader of a functional area. For example, the co-leads for the student resource sphere included a staff member (program manager) and the senior associate dean of medical education administration, while the student sphere was co-led by two students with administrative support from a staff member on the change strategy team.

    Change Consultant. Sometimes a consultant may serve as a key support to the sponsor, change process leader, and Guiding Coalition in building and carrying out the best overall change management strategy and process; acts as a sounding board and third party; educates the project community about transformation and strategies for how to proceed and achieve change targets; helps plan the change strategy, major events, communications, trainings, and meetings; assesses progress, problems, concerns, and political and cultural issues; helps facilitate change in culture, mindset, and behavior.

Our Experience: Change Consultant

Given the pointed recommendation from our students that we needed outside expertise, we first worked with Leona Hess, PhD, MSW as a consultant, and later brought her on full-time because of her work in change management, systems thinking, and antiracism. Leona's first challenge was to facilitate our executive team's ability to recognize our own interpersonal racism and biases. Our team had been working together for decades but had never deeply unearthed our assumptions about each other, our micro- and macroaggressions, and the impact of the systems within which we worked. Leona helped establish a space in which we could be vulnerable and embrace discomfort with humility and trust. The tools she introduced allowed us to gauge our readiness to take on what we knew would be a significantly more challenging task: coleading change in ever-widening concentric circles, starting with our teaching faculty and staff, students, and the larger landscape that constitutes our learning environment.

Time expected to complete activity: 1 hour.

Target audience: A select group of people who participated in Identifying the Project Community (Activity 2a) or those involved in designing the strategy or planning for change.

Purpose of the activity: To establish clear change roles and responsibilities to minimize redundancy and ensure full coverage.

Instructions:

1. During the meeting:
   a. Ask the "clarifying your roles" questions listed in Worksheet 4.2, Activity 2b.
   b. Record answers to the questions and fill out a grid in the Activity 2b: Clarifying Your Roles (Worksheet 4.2).
2. After the meeting:
   a. Individually complete the Self-Reflection Questions.

Activity 2c: Creating a Clear Case and Desired Outcome

Creating your case for change and determining the outcomes or results you want from it establishes a shared view for your project community and gives stakeholders meaning, direction, and energy for collective action. Without a clear case for change, the transformation will lack relevance, causing resistance, confusion, and insecurity. This is an important step even if your institution has already committed to becoming antiracist, especially if there has been a leadership change or existing efforts have lost momentum or direction. A case for change can always be revamped as time goes on, or if events require revisiting the need to transform, what needs to change, the big picture outcome, and who is involved.

In order to develop an effective case for change, you must consider the catalysts driving the change in your institution. Although drivers can be organized into common themes, the details of each will be unique to your institution. We recommend you address all of the drivers, as outlined by Anderson and Anderson,[1] to accurately scope out your change effort, especially when the change is transformational and aims to disrupt racism.

Our Experience: Our Case for Change

On March 5, 2018, we communicated the case for change to our medical school community with an invitation to learn more about our process and what to expect. The following passage is the communication we sent articulating our case for change. It included a short video about why we were taking a change management approach:

"The time is now. We live in a world that doesn't provide all people with the same opportunities. Just as there are social determinants of health, there are social determinants of education, social determinants of financial security, and social determinants of success in life. These persistent patterns and behaviors privilege those of us who are white, those of us who are male, those of us who have never had to worry about our immigration status, sexual orientation, or religion. They perpetuate inequalities in care for our patients, in our learning environment, and professional opportunities for our peers.

We aspire to be better than that. We want medical education and, indeed, the practice of medicine, to be the exception to that rule. Our work as staff, teachers, mentors, doctors and scientists should have equity of

opportunity as its foundation. We want medicine to be the shining example of what the rest of society should be like. We have a long road to travel before we can achieve that goal. The inequality we see all around us can change. It has to change if we are serious about transforming our culture to one that is free of racism and bias. And we can change it.

Thanks to the many students who devoted countless hours to this cause, we were able to begin an effort to address the impact of racism and bias in our medical school and our profession by launching the Racism and Bias Initiative in 2015. Since the initiative's launch we've undertaken a variety of activities and interventions related to addressing racism and bias in curricular and student affairs, admissions, and the clinical learning environment. We are now ready to move ahead. We are committed to transformational change that explicitly addresses and undoes racism and bias in all areas of the school and centers racial justice, health equity, and underrepresented voices and experiences. Our vision is to become a health system and health professions school with the most diverse workforce, providing health care and education that is free of racism and bias. We are embarking on the next phase of our initiative – the people and process side of the transformational change. We invite you to the town hall on March 20th to learn more about our strategy and how we intend to engage, prepare, equip and support individuals and medical school community as a whole."[10]

The sponsor, executive team, change strategy team, and change process lead used the following talking points to collectively reinforce the reasons why the change was necessary:
- Lives depend on it
  - Health equity gap between White patients and patients of color
  - Differential access and quality for patients of color
- Racism and bias are present – here and now
  - Persistent patterns and behaviors that privilege White students, faculty, and staff that are embedded in policies and practices
  - Persistent belief of genetic and biological view of race
  - Unequal outcomes for academic success for students of color
  - Lack of faculty of color – recruitment, retention, promotion

- Diversity and inclusion matter
  - Increases innovation and lessens biased decision-making
  - Improves both the educational experience and patient care
  - Cultivates a climate of support, equity, and inclusion
- Time to take a stand
  - Take personal responsibility
  - Commitment to wellness
  - Opportunity for personal growth and expanded awareness
  - Duty to set an example and establish best practices

All of this happened well before George Floyd was murdered. While our core principles remained very much the same, given the twin pandemics of COVID and racism our case for change continued to evolve, became more pressing, and our language became more explicit, with terms such as antiracism coming into common usage.

To create your own case for change and desired outcome, review the following drivers of change and proceed to the instructions.

The drivers of change, as described by Anderson and Anderson[1]:

- *Environmental forces.* The dynamics of the larger context within which institutions and people operate. These forces include social and demographic trends, business or economic pressures, political dynamics, government regulations, technological advances, demographic patterns, legal issues, and the natural environment.
- *Business/academic imperatives.* What the institution must do strategically to be successful, given its key stakeholders' changing needs and requirements.
- *Institutional imperatives.* What must change in the institution's structure, systems, processes, technology, resources, skill base, or staffing to realize its strategic business imperatives.
- *Cultural imperatives.* How the values, norms, or collective way of being, working, teaching, learning, and relating in the school must change to support and drive the future state (in this case, antiracism). Some change efforts are driven by a need to change the culture, such as the need for a new leadership style, more equitable decision-making processes, antiracism pedagogy, etc. If so, this driver is given more detailed attention, and ideally is still positioned in support of the institution's imperatives to change.

- *Leader and employee behavior.* Collective behavior creates and expresses an institution's culture and performance. Behavior is more than just overt actions. It describes the style, tone, or character that permeates what people do and how their way of being must change to create the new culture. Leaders and employees must choose to behave differently, individually and collectively, in order to transform the institution's culture.
- *Leader and employee mindset.* Mindset encompasses people's worldview, assumptions, beliefs, and mental models. Mindset causes people to behave as they do. Becoming aware that each of us has a mindset and that it directly impacts our feelings, decisions, actions, and results is often the critical first step in building individual and institutional awareness and willingness to change. Mindset change catalyzes and sustains new behaviors. A shift in mindset is usually required for leaders to recognize changes in environmental forces and business/academic requirements. Mindset change in employees helps them understand why the changes being asked of them are necessary, and what they must do to carry them out. Mindset is always included in transformational change efforts.

Time expected to complete activity: 1.5 hours; wordsmithing might require additional time.

Target audience: A select group of people who participated in Identifying the Project Community (Activity 2a) and/or Clarifying Your Roles (Activity 2b) or members of the change strategy team (if identified).

Purpose of the activity: To develop a clear case and desired outcome that will inform and compel people to support and adopt the change.

Instructions:

1. During the meeting:
   a. Ask the Creating a Clear Case and Designed Outcome questions listed in worksheet 4.3.
   b. Record answers to the questions and fill out a grid in the Activity 2c: Creating a Clear Case and Desired Outcome (Worksheet 4.3).
2. After the meeting:
   a. Individually complete the Self-Reflection Questions.

Activity 2d: Creating Optimal Working Relationships

Creating optimal working relationships is essential for setting the right conditions for success. We must be intentional about tending to the working relationships of those who will be involved in preparing for change and all of the phases of the change process. Toxic behaviors are normal; we cannot just get rid of them. In fact, pretending there are never toxins in a team can be viewed as a form of stonewalling. Organizational Relationship and System Coaching (ORSC) describes the four team toxins[11]:

- *Blaming.* Attacking the person rather than the behavior. For example, aggressive attack, bullying, chronic criticalness, and domination.
- *Defensiveness.* Refusing to own your own behavior, pushing back, arguing, deflection, and not being open to influence.
- *Contempt.* Cutting others down, hostile gossip, undermining, disrespect, and demeaning communication.
- *Stonewalling.* Not open to influence, cutting off communication, avoidance, uncooperativeness, passivity, disengagement, "yes men," and withholding.

There are a number of ways to resolve conflict by working with team toxins. This activity is an approach to anticipating and resolving conflict that ideally starts before major conflict has emerged in your change strategy team or other groups who are involved in preparing for change.

Time expected to complete activity: 1 hour.

Target audience: those involved in planning for change (e.g., change strategy team), even if they do not have a history of working together.

Purpose of the activity: To help those planning the change to understand and take responsibility for toxic communication patterns and to develop a conflict protocol.

Note: You will need to adapt this activity depending on the setting. For example, if you are meeting in person you can physically move around the room. If you are meeting virtually (e.g., Zoom) you will need to use the annotation feature or another mechanism to actively engage attendees.

Instructions:

1. During the meeting:
   a. Follow the team toxin discussion instructions.
   b. Ask the Conflict Protocol Questions listed later.
   c. Record answers to the questions in the Activity 2d: Creating Optimal Working Relationships (Worksheet 4.4).
2. After the meeting:
   a. Individually complete the Self-Reflection Questions.

Team Toxin Discussion

Lay a four-square out on the floor (or screen) that has a space for each of the team toxins. Label each quadrant with the definitions of the toxins. See Fig. 4.3 for an example.

Have members step into (or annotate with Zoom feature) the square they think is most commonly occupied by the team, or maybe in your institution if you have not worked together in the past. Ask the following questions:

- *What is the stance, sound, gesture of that toxin?* Keep it playful! It is fine if people identify different toxins.
- *What are the situations that bring that toxin out in the team or institution? What is the belief behind this toxin? How is it trying to be helpful?* For example, "I may act defensively because I feel misunderstood and want you to understand me." Hear from everyone. Notice what toxin grids are not occupied, and ask about them. Ask each attendee to go to the one they most often employ. What situations bring that toxin out in them?

Develop a conflict protocol on how your group will handle conflict when it arises.

Conflict Protocol Questions

Conflict is a signal that something is trying to happen. When handled skillfully it can lead to constructive change. Toxic conflict can paralyze a team, induce absenteeism, and reduce the effectiveness to lead change.

While you answer these questions you may find yourself repeating something as you answer. The repetition is

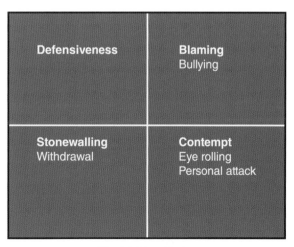

Fig. 4.3 Team Toxins

pointing to something important, such as patterned behavior.

Keep the conflict protocol visible throughout the change process phases and revisit the protocol when necessary. If new people join the various change roles, we recommend introducing them to the protocol or revising if needed.

REFERENCES

1. Anderson LA, Anderson D. *The Change Leader's Roadmap: How to Navigate Your Organization's Transformation.* Vol. 384. Hoboken, NJ: John Wiley & Sons; 2010.
2. Dorman PT. *From Command and Control to Modern Approaches to Leadership.* HealthManagement; 2023. https://healthmanagement.org/c/icu/issuearticle/from-command-and-control-to-modern-approaches-to-leadership.
3. Dobbin F, Kalev A. Why doesn't diversity training work? the challenge for industry and academia. *Anthropol Now.* 2018;10(2):48-55. doi:10.1080/19428200.2018.1493182.
4. Anderson P. *Building a Culture of Accountability. How to Build a Culture of Accountability to Promote Racial Equity in Your Organization.* Stanford Social Innovation Review; 2021. https://ssir.org/articles/entry/building_a_culture_of_accountability.
5. Wells R. *Self-Assessment Tool: Anti-Racism.* United Way of Addison County. https://unitedwayaddisoncounty.org/client_media/files/ReneeWellsAntiRacismSelfAssessmentTool.pdf.
6. Puget Sound Cohort, Race Forward. *Accountability Principles - Facing Race: A National Conference.* Accountability Principles; 2019. https://facingrace.raceforward.org/sites/default/files/RaceForward_PugetSoundCohort_FINAL.pdf.
7. Souza T. *Responding to Microaggressions in The Classroom: Taking Action.* Faculty Focus; 2018. https://www.facultyfocus.com/articles/effective-classroom-management/responding-to-microaggressions-in-the-classroom.
8. INCITE! Women of Color Against Violence! *Community Accountability Factsheet.* https://transformharm.org/ca_resource/community-accountability-factsheet.
9. Buzan T, Buzan B. *The Mind Mapping Book; Radiant Thinking - The Major Evolution in Human Thought.* London: BBC Books; 1993.
10. Anand S, Butts G. *Town Hall Meeting - Racism and Bias Initiative.* DropBox; 2018. https://www.dropbox.com/s/8s2all2bkld9zsn/RBI%20Town%20Hall%20Communication.pdf?dl=0.
11. CRR Global. *About ORSC.* 2022. https://crrglobal.com/about/orsc/.

Phase 3: Creating a Climate for Change

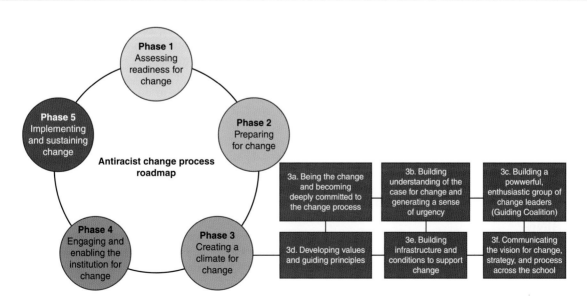

MOVING INTO MIDSTREAM CHANGE

The goal of phase 3 is to create a climate for change. It might seem counterintuitive, but there are critically important steps that come before implementing the change. You might be feeling "fix it" pressure from students, colleagues, and/or leadership, or you might find this phase a distraction from the "real" work. Remember, it is when we leap ahead to implementation without laying the groundwork that most change efforts flounder.[1,2] Make no mistake, implementation is important and is going to happen, but it is the *last* stage of the change process. Most implementation problems can be avoided by getting the upstream and midstream stages right.

Before jumping into phase 3, let's first define a *climate for change*. The climate of an organization consists of the moment-by-moment interactions that people experience and interpret in an emotional context.[3] Climate creates a state of mind. It is what is felt when we enter a room or space, and it can change from day to day, from meeting to meeting. Climate is our attitude and it is based on our perceptions. Climate is the first thing that improves when a positive change is made. Thus the goal is to intentionally create a climate for antiracist transformational change before we implement the actual change. From a change management perspective, creating a climate means tending to the people side of change by preparing your project community, or stakeholders, to be emotionally ready for transformation and willing to embark on the process together.

Drawing from the work of Kotter, and Anderson and Anderson,[1,4] this chapter will outline the six steps for creating a climate for change. As in the previous chapter, we will provide detailed instructions on how to execute the activities, and where applicable we will share our experiences related to the change process. First, we invite those who are involved in creating a climate for change to consider employing antiracist practices while completing these activities. In the next section, we have outlined an antiracist practice that is aligned with and can enhance your ability to create a climate for antiracist change.

ANTIRACIST PRACTICE: POWER SHARING

Power sharing means widening—and shifting—the circle of people involved in transformational change, and centering people who are most impacted by inequities.[5]

In organizations there are people who hold formal and informal power. Formal power is given to someone based on their title or position. People carry informal power if they have personal or organizational influence as a result of their experience, expertise, personality, ability to persuade, unearned privilege, or because they have strong relationships with decision-makers and peers. Power, whether formal or informal, can manifest in how decisions are made, which people and networks are involved in the decisions, how problems and solutions are framed, and what ideas are even considered. Power comes in the form of resources, access to decision-making, alliances and networks, and the dominant narratives that are enforced and reinforced.

When facilitating meetings to achieve the six steps for creating a climate for change, consider taking the following actions to address the power dynamics at play[6]:

- *Assume power dynamics are always present in your meetings.* Design your activity or Guiding Coalition meeting agenda to include multiple voices and perspectives. You can encourage people from the change strategy team to lead and participate, especially if they have less power in the institution because of role, positional status, race, gender, or other factors. Encourage people with traditional forms of formal power to do more listening than speaking. Pay attention to who is participating and contributing to the conversation. Name power dynamics when they happen and ask for perspectives that have not been expressed.

- *Build a culture of collaboration.* Think of the phase activities and Guiding Coalition meetings as an opportunity to build relationships, design good processes, and counteract unhealthy uses of power. We encourage you to build an agenda that allows people to first interact on a human basis. Start with opportunities for people to do a check-in and share how their day or week is going, or to learn more about each other on a personal level by answering icebreaker questions. You can also create openings for people to feel heard and noticed (kudos or shout outs), and to experience a sense of belonging and interconnectedness. The goal is to encourage honesty and vulnerability, and to set expectations for when it is necessary to call people "in" or "out." For more information about how to set up these conditions, use the "Calling In and Calling Out Guide."[7,8]

You can also design activities and Guiding Coalition meetings to allow for maximum creativity. Employ more creative or lateral thinking by brainstorming, forming associations with the topic at hand, and questioning the status quo to find solutions.

- *Openly discuss power during activities and Guiding Coalition meetings.* What would be the benefits of shared power? Remind members that power is not a finite resource; it can be infinite, expanded, and shared among people and leaders. Prompt them to explore how they can share power *with* each other instead of power *over* each other. Make a list of meeting agreements that the group will use to share power. Ask people to monitor the agreements and be brave enough to intervene if people are not practicing them. Make a list of 'power *over*' moves so people learn the behaviors that reinforce dominant voices and exclude others. Have people take mental note of who is speaking the most and who is not. How are they behaving at the table? How are their priorities, assets, and skills driving the discussion?

- *Remember that power is a social construct.* We can design spaces where individuals and groups experience their own and others' power differently. Be proactive about ways to amplify the power of people who are typically at the margins of the conversation. Challenge the group to pay at least as much attention to the expertise that comes from lived experience as from formal theories and data. Flip questions on their head by asking how you can do things differently instead of how you can work within given boundaries. Ensure that people who are affected by racism are at the center of the conversation and have meaningful roles in the work over time.

- *Use your role intentionally and thoughtfully if you are the Guiding Coalition meeting facilitator.* Do not dominate the discussion. Do not come up with all the ideas. Stay as impartial as possible, even though you can never truly be completely neutral. If you want to contribute an idea or experience, tell the group you are switching from facilitator role to express your view as an individual, and then step back into your facilitator role. Examine who gets to facilitate meetings and who does not. Meeting facilitators can change the outcome of the meeting based on how they design and run it. Rotating facilitation and supporting people who want to learn how to facilitate meetings distributes power and makes meetings more dynamic.

SIX STEPS FOR CREATING A CLIMATE FOR CHANGE

As in the previous chapter, these six steps do not need to be completed in order, although we have scaffolded the activities to build on one another. We recommend that you treat these steps as iterative and continue to update or refine them as new information becomes available. You should carefully consider who needs to inform each of the steps and what voices and perspectives are needed.

Being the Change and Becoming Deeply Committed to the Change Process

The first step is introspective. Everyone creating a climate for change is encouraged to take a moment to pause, self-reflect, and debrief as a group. Check in with yourself to ensure you are 'being the change' and becoming deeply committed to the change process.

Building Understanding of the Case for Change and Generating a Sense of Urgency

The second step involves beginning to build your project community's understanding of the case for change and generating a sense of urgency. This is done through kick-off communications that align your project community with transformational change. This step involves utilizing the case for change (Activity 2c) and project community map (Activity 2a) that were developed in phase 2.

Building and Supporting a Powerful, Enthusiastic Group of Change Leaders

The third step requires building a powerful, enthusiastic group of change leaders, also known as the *Guiding Coalition*. This will broaden the depth and breadth of your change process.

Developing Values and Guiding Principles

The fourth step involves developing the overarching vision, values, and guiding principles that will align the role of the Guiding Coalition with the change process.

Building Infrastructure and Conditions to Support Change

The fifth step allows the Guiding Coalition to identify (1) the infrastructure and conditions needed to support change in order to secure resources and (2) areas where they can proactively build in support.

Communicating the Vision for Change, Strategy, and Process Across the School

The sixth step circles back to the project community by sharing the vision for change, strategy, and change process.

PHASE 3 ACTIVITIES AND INSTRUCTIONS

The six activities outlined in this section are designed for different target audiences. We recommend completing the first two activities with the *change strategy team* or others who are involved in creating a climate for change. The remaining four activities should be completed by the Guiding Coalition.

Activity 3a: Being the Change and Becoming Deeply Committed to the Change Process

Anderson and Anderson suggest that our "mindset, emotion, and behavior are intricately linked and interact with one another as an interconnected system that is referred to as one's way of being."[1] For example, the mindset that "change should be fast and painless" when complex, long-term change is actually required, may cause you to be impatient and frustrated at the slow pace. Behaviorally, as Anderson and Anderson point out, you may become controlling, domineering, and autocratic. While mindsets might cause emotions and behaviors, the combination of all three is the source of one's way of being.

When embarking on transformational change in a complex adaptive system, it is important to consider your way of being. For example, what are your mindsets, emotions, and behaviors related to the change process? How do you come across to others? How do you know?

In addition to your way of being, there is also the way in which you walk the talk of change. Anderson and Anderson suggest that "talk" denotes your vision of desired behaviors, and "walk" denotes the behaviors and actions you actually model. When these are not aligned and you consistently say one thing and do another, it establishes a predictable path that leads to distrust, increases resistance among stakeholders, and damages all hope of building commitment for the transformation.[1,8] Walking the talk of change essentially means leading from the "way of being" that is consistent with your desired culture and role modeling it into existence. Of course, you will also need to align this with systems, structures, processes, and technology, but we will come to that in the next phase.

For now, consider how you might align with and commit to the change process. What does that look like? Walking the talk does not mean that you need to be perfect all of the time. Anderson and Anderson suggest that mistakes and gaps are expected and quite acceptable as long as you do three things: (1) acknowledge your incongruent behavior to yourself and those it impacts; (2) make amends as appropriate; and (3) become more consistent in your talk and walk over time.

Time expected to complete activity: Complete individually in one week and debrief as a group (~ 1 hour).

Target audience: The change strategy team or anyone who is involved in creating a climate for change.

Purpose of the activity: To identify personal habitual reactions and patterns, and assess the ways in which the change strategy team is walking the talk.

Instructions:

1. The personal daily log:
   a. Use the Personal Daily Log in Worksheet 5.1 for 1 week.
   b. During the day, record when you react to external situations and find yourself notably "Centered and Effective" (positive) in your reaction or "Reacted in a Way You Would Like to Change" (negative).
   c. In just a couple of days, analyze your patterns and notice the situations that activate similar mental, emotional and physical states, behaviors, actions, and results. The goal is to become more familiar with your internal states and recognize them more quickly so you can either course-correct or reinforce them.
2. Once you have completed the Personal Daily Log Worksheet 5.1, reflect on the Becoming the Change Questions, as outlined below.
3. After completing, debrief with members of the change strategy team. We recommend scheduling a meeting to debrief the questions and discuss any next steps.
4. After the debrief meeting, individually complete the Self-Reflection Questions and follow up on any action items.

Becoming the Change Questions:

1. What did you learn about your way of being? Consider the patterns emerging across the columns.
2. How might your way of being influence: (1) what you see in the antiracist transformation, (2) your internal experiences with the change, (3) your decisions,

(4) your impact on others, and (5) your change results or outcomes?

3. At this time, what personal transformational work might you focus on? What does that "work" look like for you?

4. How do you know when you are walking the talk of antiracist change? What are the desired behaviors, actions, and relationships?

5. What do you need, from yourself and others, in order to deeply commit to the change process?

6. How can you hold yourself accountable? What does that look like?

Postdebrief Self-Reflection Questions:

Self-reflection is an important antiracist practice and aspect of the process towards transformation. After completing Activity 3a, spend time self-reflecting on the following questions:

1. Did anything surprise you about the debrief meeting?

2. Is there anything that needs follow up or more attention at this time?

Activity 3b: Building Understanding of the Case for Change and Generating a Sense of Urgency

During this step, the project community will build a deeper understanding of the case for antiracist change and the process for getting there. If you have already developed a communication strategy related to your antiracist and/or diversity, equity, and inclusion (D/E/I) efforts, we encourage you to use this activity as a way of assessing if you have included the components that align your communications with transformational change.

The kickoff communication is your formal declaration to the project community that an antiracist transformation is underway. This is different from a declaration or announcement of an antiracist or D/E/I strategic plan. Its content, tone, and delivery methods have a significant impact on how people respond, and right-size their expectations of the impending challenge of transformation. It sets the stage for how institutional leaders such as the deans and C-suite will be perceived as leaders of this transformation, how much commitment to change exists within the project community, and whether stakeholders believe in the overall change strategy. Make no mistake, this initial communication about the case for change and details about the change strategy is one of the most important opportunities you

will have to mobilize the project community through open dialogue, and potentially recruit members to the Guiding Coalition.

As plenty of medical schools have already launched task forces and committees to create strategic plans for addressing racism, many people have already received communications about what might change and the desired goals. It is important that you build on these initial communications to ensure you are effectively introducing change that is transformational, as well as the process for getting there. For some this might be a paradigm shift from the traditional linear thinking that tells us to identify a problem, fix it, and move to the next problem. This type of communication can also present an opportunity to reinvigorate members of your project community who might be skeptical of the current state or feel as if there has not been movement towards real or tangible change.

When designing your transformational change kickoff communication strategy, remember to address three important people dynamics. Anderson and Anderson suggest that people's initial reactions to the transformation may be colored by[1,8]:

1. Their concern for what the change means to them personally. Be prepared to identify WIIFM (what's in it for me) for different stakeholder groups across your project community. For example, what does it mean to be antiracist, on a day-to-day basis, in my role and function? What does it mean for our class, group, or team? What does it mean for the strategic direction of the institution?

2. Their attachment to the status quo. Even when people want to see change, they are often more attached to how things are or have been over time. This is even true when it comes to addressing racism or other systems of oppression. Remember that we have been trained to rationalize and adapt to whatever the current reality is.

3. The emotions they still have about past changes in which they were adversely affected. Many of our institutions operate on a "flavor of the month" approach, which shifts priorities when new hot topics arise. Often this leaves people feeling change fatigue, with minimal confidence in the direction the institution is headed because there will always be something new to divert their attention. We have seen numerous examples of this when institutions react to social injustices by prioritizing new initiatives, task forces, committees,

and plans, with minimal accountability to demonstrate long-term impact or improvement.

Transformational change kickoff communications may include any of the following content:

- Who is leading the change and in what capacity; who are the sponsors and the role of the Guiding Coalition?
- The case for change, including the story of the *seven drivers of change*.
- Scope of the change and why it is transformational, including the mindset and cultural imperatives for antiracist change.
- Conditions for success.
- Expectations for people's engagement and commitment.
- Other components based on existing communications and strategic plans, roadmaps, and actions.

We recommend creating a "cheat sheet" to mitigate against information overload and feeling "lost" in the change process. The change strategy team can create a communications cheat sheet that includes all of the content of the kickoff communications. The cheat sheet can provide: (1) templated text where people can cut and paste to decrease the time it takes to craft certain communications; (2) talking points about the change process to reinforce messaging and increase the speaker's confidence; (3) common language so people receive consistent messaging, appear unified in their messaging, and demonstrate collaboration; and (4) timeline of the various communications that go out after broader emails or blogs, thus helping you better plan your roadmap activities.

It is important to note that there is not one approach to kickoff communications. Your communications will be tailored and responsive to what is happening in your institution. To help provide guidance, in Table 5.1 we have adapted the effective kickoff communications components[1] to illustrate our approach.

TABLE 5.1	**Effective Transformational Change Kickoff Communications Example**		
Owner/Sender	**Action**	**Description**	**Our Experience**
Sponsor(s), change strategy team, and executive team	Share initial communication.	Through numerous large in-person or virtual group meetings. More than one person speaks to enliven the delivery. Speakers share the case for change and change strategy, request input for the vision of the future, and encourage people to participate in generating the shared vision by joining the Guiding Coalition.	In the previous chapter we shared our initial communications, which included an email with a whiteboard video outlining the transformational change management approach. We then followed up the communications with a large in-person town hall that revealed the vision and showcased brief presentations from the Dean, the Dean for Medical Education, and the senior associate deans of the functional areas of the medical school. Each presenter discussed where they were at on their own person growth and commitment to antiracism and outlined how their functional areas will be part of the change and participate in the Guiding Coalition. There was an opportunity for questions and answers. The audience was invited to sign up ("open call") to be a member of the Guiding Coalition.

TABLE 5.1   Effective Transformational Change Kickoff Communications Example—cont'd

Owner/Sender	Action	Description	Our Experience
Sponsor(s) and change strategy team	Discuss initial communication with groups across the project community.	Follow up with a series of town hall meetings, web discussions, or blogs that cascade throughout the project community to openly discuss what was said in the initial communications, reiterating the facts and addressing perceptions and fears. During this time it is critical to listen and respond to questions. A short time is provided between sessions or events to allow stakeholders to talk and post about what they heard.	After our town hall we launched various blog posts and content on our ChangeNow website. This allowed us to publicly display our case for change, timeline of the process, recording of the town hall, results from the post–town hall survey, and a feedback and comments section that we later used to inform communications. Here is an example of a blog post that was created to address the top nine questions post–town hall: https://changenow.icahn.mssm.edu/town-hall-nine-questions-nine-answers/
Sponsor(s) and change strategy team	Discuss reactions and identify potential Guiding Coalition members.	Facilitating breakout conversations (or online blogs) about general reactions or key issues allows for active involvement by all stakeholders. Major messages from the breakout groups are brought back to the larger group (or main online platform) for presentation to, and response by, the change strategy team and sponsors. Each meeting is concluded by describing opportunities to be part of the Guiding Coalition, to create an informal network that will be asked for input, and to represent each functional area's interests as the transformation is planned and implemented.	The POD (our change strategy team) identified existing group meetings (student groups, committees of staff, course and clerkship directors, etc.) where we elicited general reactions to the change strategy and identified key issues. We were intentional about listening, as opposed to responding, and being transparent about what we knew, what we did not know, and what would unfold as the Guiding Coalition embarked on its process.
Guiding Coalition members and sphere leads; change strategy team; and executive team	Facilitate team discussions.	Facilitate discussions in their functional areas across the school/project community using blogs about the transformation, its implications for each functional area, and for individual members. The functional areas are tasked with identifying what is already happening, likely barriers to the effort, and their desired future state.	Each of the Guiding Coalition spheres convened people in their functional area to answer these questions: What is the terrain in which we work and/or learn in our sphere? Who are we, and what are we becoming? What are our big picture needs or gaps as it relates to our future vision? With that data, we created a blog post to illustrate the diverse landscape of the project community.

Continued

TABLE 5.1	Effective Transformational Change Kickoff Communications Example—cont'd		
Owner/Sender	**Action**	**Description**	**Our Experience**
Sponsors, executive team	Deploy a mass communication status report of the transformation effort.	Mass communication vehicle that provides a current status report of the transformation effort. It highlights actions taken and outcomes produced as a direct result of the rollout, and input from stakeholders. Share stories about how various stakeholders have had insights or breakthroughs or have mobilized action central to the transformation's success.	Early on in the process, we provided updates in person, by email, and by blog posts on the ChangeNow website. As time went on, the Guiding Coalition started to host quarterly interactive meetings where anyone could come to learn about the progress and challenges. Starting in 2021, we created a "year in review" report that we shared with the project community. We also sent out monthly "Action Updates" newsletters via Mailchimp (these archives can be accessed) and posted on ChangeNow.

Time expected to complete activity: 1.5 hours per part.

Target audience: The change strategy team or anyone who is involved in creating a climate for change.

Purpose of the activity: To develop an effective kickoff communication strategy that builds understanding of the case for change across your project community.

Instructions:

There are two parts related to this activity. Part 1 helps you develop kickoff communications and part 2 narrows the focus on the sponsor role. For both parts we recommend setting up meetings with the target audience to complete.

Part 1: Planning Kickoff Communications

Using Table 5.1 as a guide, fill out Worksheet 5.2 to develop your initial transformational change kickoff communications.

We recommend using the *five levels of communication* as outlined in Table 5.2 as you think through your communication style and method or vehicle. The five levels begin where most people end their communication efforts: sharing information. It goes on to four subsequent levels in the communication process: building understanding, identifying implications, gaining commitment, and altering behavior.

The goal is to develop communications that include multiple opportunities for stakeholder groups to hear the case for change; talk and think about it; formulate their questions; and have their concerns addressed. The intervals between conversations will enable stakeholders to discuss their concerns with others, which in turn will generate more questions. Eventually, the process will generate greater understanding and acceptance. Honoring the "process" of effective communication will help ensure a successful kickoff to your transformation and build the required critical mass of commitment and intention.[1,8]

Part 2: Engaging Sponsors

As you start to plan your transformational kickoff communications, determine what aspects of the change process will require assistance and support from your sponsor(s). You can utilize the Sponsor Roadmap Worksheet 5.3 as a planning tool to prepare, equip, and support your sponsors effectively.

A sponsor roadmap outlines the tasks and engagement strategies your sponsors need to fulfill their role in the kickoff communications and beyond. These tasks should be centered around the sponsor's engagement with the change strategy team, other senior leaders, and others directly affected by the change. By coming to the sponsors with an organized list of tasks they need to assist with, they will gain a better sense of how much support they will need to give to the effort, and provide transparent accountability.

TABLE 5.2   Five Levels of Communication

	Style	Media/Vehicles	Reaction When Achieved
1. **Information sharing**	Telling; one way	Lecture, presentation, memo, broadcast, video, digital signage	"Thank you for sharing."
2. **Building understanding**	Dialogue; two way; exploring and answering listener-generated questions	Small groups or breakouts; facilitated questions and answers; blogs; polling (e.g., Poll Everywhere or Slido); virtual session; web-based notice board (Padlet)	"Having explored my concerns and tested this, I now understand the focus of the change and why it is needed."
3. **Identifying implications**	Introspection; discussing with others what this means to you and the institution; multidirectional	Group interactive discussions ranging from multilevel, large, or small group discussions; most relevant exploration done with teams, groups, or classes and immediate supervisor or faculty; web-based notice board (Padlet) or discussion boards; storytelling; Conversation Café; Open Space Technology; World Café	"I get it! This change means X for my department/team/class and Z for me and my job/role."
4. **Commitment**	Sorting out inner feelings and choices; may require time and multiple returns to the discussion; focused on both internal and external commitments	Alone time for personal introspection or "talk time" with trusted colleagues or classmates; opportunity to readdress issues with classmates, colleagues, direct supervisor, and/or sponsor of the change	"I personally want this change to succeed, and I am willing to ensure that it does. I see that others and our institution's leaders feel the same way."
5. **Altering behavior**	Demonstrating new behavior; may require training, feedback mechanisms, and coaching over time to ensure that the behaviors stick	Training, coaching relationships; opportunities for practice and learning	"I am learning the new behaviors and skills required for this change to succeed, and I'm open to receiving your feedback and coaching to keep improving."

Adapted from Anderson LA, Anderson D. *The Change Leader's Roadmap: How to Navigate Your Organization's Transformation.* Vol. 384. Hoboken, NJ: John Wiley & Sons; 2010.

Activity 3c: Building a Powerful Enthusiastic Group of Change Leaders (Guiding Coalition)

A traditional organizational hierarchy is the typical operating system found in all of our institutions. Although this system allows us to meet the daily demands of running a medical school or health system, it is not designed for an environment where change can become the norm, especially antiracist transformation. John Kotter advocates for a new system: a second, more agile, network-like structure that operates in concert with the hierarchy to create what he calls a "dual operating system,"[5] (Fig. 5.1).

A dual operating system allows institutions to run more smoothly and accelerates systemic change. Kotter suggests that this is not an either/or approach; it is both/and.[4] The two systems operate in concert and must be linked. If all we do is try to manage the hierarchy, we have no hope of developing the innovations that are needed for transformational change. On the other hand, if all we do is focus on the network-like structure, the innovations will never see the light of day or will be met with lots of resistance. The key is to do both.

The network-like structure that Kotter is talking about is called a Guiding Coalition. As discussed in Chapter 4, a Guiding Coalition is a group of people working together to influence outcomes on a specific

The hierarchy and network form a dual operating system

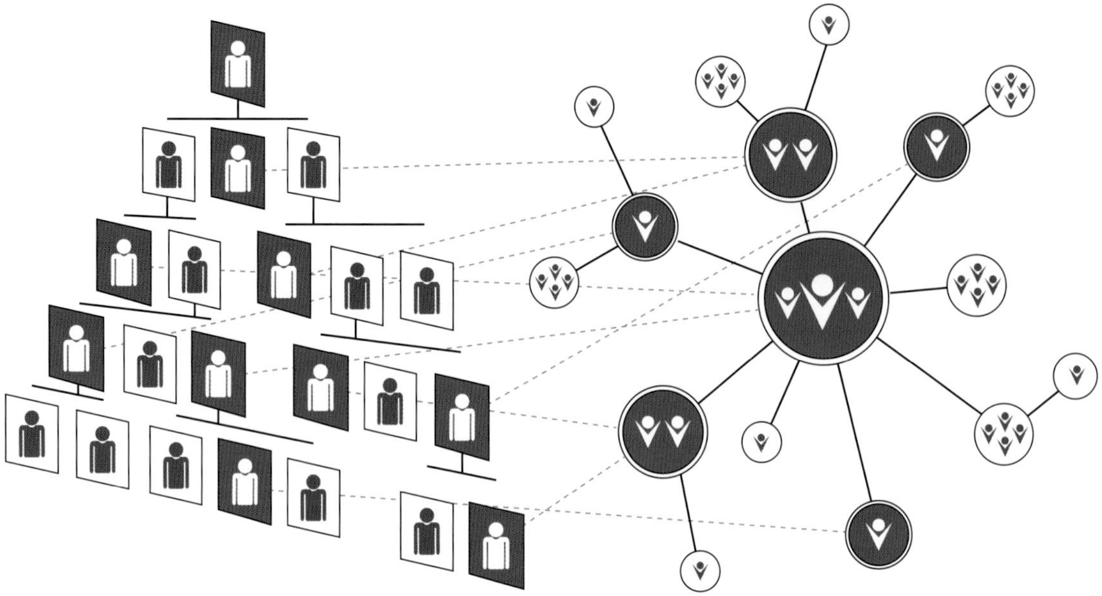

Fig. 5.1 Dual Operating System. (From Kotter J. *Accelerate: Building strategic agility for a faster-moving world.* Boston, MA: Harvard Business School Press; 2014; The Dual Operating System concet, John. P. Kotter, XLR8.)

issue. The coalition is useful for accomplishing a broad range of goals that reach beyond the capacity of any individual, team, or silo. Members of the coalition are a powerful, enthusiastic group of change leaders who develop new innovations and put them into effect to transform an institution.

In this case, the Guiding Coalition will be responsible for setting direction for the antiracism transformational change. They will oversee the change initiatives or actions, identify options and make decisions about where energy and resources should be focused, determine how to hold people accountable, manage resistance, and muster support, buy-in, and resources from stakeholders and other parts of their institution.

Generally speaking, there are four qualities of an effective Guiding Coalition[4]:

1. *Positional power.* Enough key players on board so that those left out cannot block progress.
2. *Expertise.* All relevant points of view should be represented so that informed and intelligent decisions can be made and a short feedback loop can be established to develop strategies or test activities. Members should bring with them a variety of unique

characteristics that contribute to the effort. This might vary by skills, lived experiences, identities, perspectives, and networking abilities.

3. *Credibility.* The group should be seen and respected by all so that the group's pronouncements will be taken seriously by others.
4. *Leadership.* The group should have enough proven leaders (this includes all levels of leadership, management and nonmanagement) that are able to drive the change process.

Membership Expectation

- Members use their day-to-day function/role and respective stakeholder groups to increase awareness of the change initiative and adoption of the change process roadmap.
- Contribute energy and skills by collaborating on change projects or actions that will accelerate antiracism change in a specific sphere, attending monthly meetings, and working between meetings.
- Increase personal awareness, knowledge, and ability in order to address racism in systemic policies and practices that have generated an imbalance

in power and privilege in the learning and work environment.

Membership Criteria

- Value diversity comprehensively, including race, ethnicity, gender, religion, sexual orientation, ability and disability, age, and other factors that shape creative perspectives and professional experiences.
- Demonstrate a high commitment to ending racism and inequities.
- Be open minded and willing to approach problems with an awareness that one's own perspective is not always the only valid perspective.
- Have personal goals and talents that are aligned with the antiracism transformation agenda and vision.
- Demonstrate a desire to transform "why we cannot" into "how we can."
- Affect change through actions big and small.
- Motivation to lead from where you sit.

Membership Commitment

It is important to be transparent about membership commitment. People should be aware of what they are signing up for prior to attending the Guiding Coalition. Table 5.3 outlines *examples* of membership commitments that can be shared during recruitment.

Building a Guiding Coalition

Recruitment can take on different forms. You can invite members who meet the criteria and who have the ability to commit to the Guiding Coalition. You may also choose to conduct an open application process. We recommend doing both. We have found that there are folks, like frontline staff, who typically are not offered these types of opportunities and who are interested and able to contribute powerful insights and energy to the Guiding Coalition's purpose.

The goal is to ensure full representation from all functional areas of the project community. No group should be left out.

Our Experience: The Racism and Bias Initiative's Guiding Coalition

We established a group of enthusiastic and influential change leaders called the Guiding Coalition. The Guiding Coalition was made up of members from every constituency in the MD program. The small, less diverse, and less representative group of MD program leaders who started this journey joined the Guiding Coalition, but handed the reins over to the larger group, in essence sharing power, privilege, and decision-making. When determining who should be on the Guiding Coalition, we centered marginalized voices and considered positional power, social influence, expertise,

TABLE 5.3 **Examples of Guiding Coalition Membership Commitments**	
Serve a 1-year term.	Membership can be extended beyond 1 year based on change projects and actions, level of commitment, coalition needs, etc.
Attend in-person monthly 90-minute meetings.	These meetings may include professional development opportunities, check ins, updates, troubleshooting, eliminating obstacles, and managing resistance.
Work in-between monthly meetings to accomplish tasks related to change projects or actions.	Could include, but is not limited to: meeting and planning with staff, faculty, and leadership; developing the right vision, objectives, or targets for change in your sphere; communicating and building awareness and desire to change; researching best practices; developing tools and materials; anchoring new approaches deep in the culture; applying change management methodology to day-to-day work.
Track change projects and actions in your functional area (sphere) and report back to Guiding Coalition via email.	A template will be provided to track and report on project or action status, wins, barriers, etc.
Attend any scheduled workshops related to the change effort (e.g., unconscious bias).	All members will have an opportunity to deepen their knowledge and skills.

credibility, and leadership ability. There was an open call for members and anyone, from front-line staff to institutional leadership, could join. We were also maximally flexible with participation, allowing people who joined initially to change their mind and step out, late comers to join when they felt ready to commit, and active members to step out temporarily when other priorities (examples included accreditation, student crises, pandemic pressures, etc.) pulled them away.

Our Guiding Coalition is now made up of seven spheres that represent the functional areas of the medical education program as well as a sphere dedicated to the program itself, which we define in Fig. 5.2. Each of the spheres has a direct impact on stakeholder groups and as a result promotes broad-based action across the project community. Members work to adopt the change management methodology; use their day-to-day function/role to increase awareness of the change initiatives; contribute their energy and skills to collaborate by attending monthly meetings; and working between meetings on change targets or actions that accelerate change both within their respective spheres and across the school.

Our Guiding Coalition is also committed to increasing personal awareness, knowledge, and ability so that we can integrate antiracist practices in the learning and work environment. Members participate in workshops and other learning opportunities at least quarterly.

Four Components to Building a Guiding Coalition

There are four components to building a powerful and enthusiastic Guiding Coalition: designing a team alliance; conducting appreciative inquiry interviews; assessing change attributes; and uncovering change characteristics. We recommend identifying two people to cofacilitate each component during the first few Guiding Coalition meetings. The Coalition must invest this time upfront to ensure its ability to build cohesiveness and gain a shared understanding of the type of change it is undertaking.

Component 1: Designing the Team Alliance

Time expected to complete activity: 1 hour.

Target audience: Guiding Coalition members.

Purpose of the activity: This activity allows participants to clearly visualize and gain an understanding of the team's intentions and agreements in order to create an environment for change and establish how members will hold each other accountable.

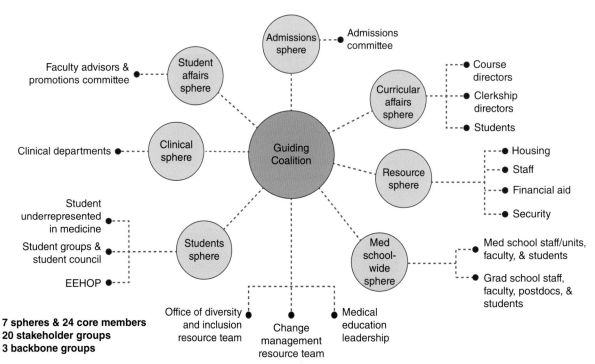

7 spheres & 24 core members
20 stakeholder groups
3 backbone groups

Fig. 5.2 Guiding Coalition

Instructions:

Prior to designing the team alliance, choose two Guiding Coalition members to serve as the scribe and timekeeper.

At the outset it is important for Guiding Coalition members to begin to build rapport and create alliances. This activity establishes the foundational platform upon which all other work will occur. In designing the team alliance, you want to help the Coalition members find alignment on the purpose and set ground rules for the Coalition, taking the first steps in consciously determining their culture and being responsible to each other for maintaining that culture.

The team alliance has three components: (1) creating culture or atmosphere; (2) creating shared responsibility; and (3) behavioral agreements.[9]

- *Creating the culture or atmosphere.* Use the following prompts and record answers on newsprint or whiteboard (visible to all members).
  1. What is the culture/atmosphere you want to create together? How will you know when you have established that?
  2. What would help the Guiding Coalition flourish?
  3. How do you want to be together when things gets difficult? What kind of speech, behaviors, and attitudes do you want to embody? How will you know when you have achieved that? Are there any antiracist practices to employ?
- *Creating shared responsibility.*
  1. What can each of you be counted on for?
  2. What's your commitment to one another?
- *Behavioral agreements.*
  1. What are the ground rules around conflict, decision-making, and other team behaviors? Are there any antiracist practices to employ?

All three parts should be visible at every Guiding Coalition meeting and revisited when needed. You might need to consolidate answers and streamline so that it's easier to use. The Guiding Coalition facilitators can use all three parts as a technique to name and address the behaviors and actions happening during meetings. Encourage members of the Coalition to hold each other accountable and not just rely on the facilitators.

Component 2: Conducting an Appreciative Inquiry Interview

Time expected to complete: 1 hour.
Target audience: Guiding Coalition members.
Purpose of the activity: The purpose of this activity is to enhance the Coalition's openness to change by deliberately working from accounts of a "positive change core."

Instructions[10]:

Appreciative interviewing, a discovery process that builds on appreciative inquiry principles, can be used to uncover shared themes and values.[11] This process can help Guiding Coalition members understand how they interact and connect with one another, and what they can accomplish when they are at their best. Appreciative interview questions are designed to collect rich qualitative information in the form of stories that carry a wealth of meaning, and sometimes a powerful emotional charge.

- Divide the Guiding Coalition into pairs. If there is an odd number of members, having one trio is okay (be sure to allow a few extra minutes for this group).
- Distribute Worksheet 5.4 to each member. Have the pairs interview each other (about 10–15 minutes/person), asking the questions exactly as they are worded on the worksheet. In each pair, one person at a time should conduct the whole interview and summarize what they heard, before moving to the other interview.
- After the pairs are finished, reconvene as a larger group and have someone from each pair share their summaries. As the facilitator, capture themes on the flipchart or whiteboard.
- Once themes are captured, have participants reflect on the themes and what they might reveal about the Guiding Coalition.

Component 3: Assessing Change Attributes

This exercise can be facilitated by itself or with the Uncovering Change Characteristics activity (Component 4).

Time expected to complete: 1 hour debrief; send survey at least one week prior to meeting.
Target audience: Guiding Coalition members.
Purpose of the activity: The purpose of this exercise is to assess your project community/institution's culture, values, and capacity for change. For an institution to get to where it wants, it must first understand where it is, as well as its current strengths and weaknesses.
Instructions:

- Create a survey with a 5-point scale that serves to measure your project community/institution's adaptability, capacity, and "baggage." Use the statements noted below when developing your assessment.
- Prior to the meeting, instruct Coalition members to rank each of the statements.
- In the meeting, share the data and spend some time discussing where people ranked a few of the

statements. Focus on similarities/overlap and outliers/conflicts.

- Conclude the meeting by exploring how this data might inform the Guiding Coalition's approach and work over the next 6 to 12 months.

Sample survey/assessment questions:

Use a 5-point scale: "On a scale of 1 to 5 with 1 being … and 5 being …" or "Strongly agree, agree, neutral, disagree, strongly disagree."

Adaptability to change: value system and culture:

- The (institution/medical school/health system)'s vision is clear.
- The vision aligns with that of our change effort (antiracist transformational change).
- The vision is embraced/upheld by members of the (institution/school/health system).
- The vision is relevant.
- The vision is sustainable.
- There is trust among all members of (name of school or other identifier).
- The institution responds in a timely fashion to feedback.
- The institution has means of receiving feedback.

Capacity for change: how much more the institution can absorb:

- The institution has team-coaching/team-teaching models or dynamics.
- The institution has effective communication among all departments/functional areas.
- The institution has ample resources to enact the changes.
- The institution has change-making power appropriately distributed among its members.
- The institution has innovators or risk takers at every level.

Residual effects of past changes; past failures may result in "baggage":

- The institution has a history of significant policy changes.
- The institution has a system of accountability.
- The institution has a significant sense of belonging.
- The institution supports and protects its members.
- The institution's higher administration has a means of receiving feedback.
- The institution has ways of retaining effective members and/or has systems for professional upward mobility.

Component 4: Uncovering Change Characteristics

This activity can be facilitated by itself or with the Assessing Change Attributes activity (Component 3).

Time expected to complete: 1 hour.

Target audience: Guiding Coalition members.

Purpose of the Activity: The purpose of this exercise is to assist the Guiding Coalition in understanding what transformational change might look like for them, as individuals and as a group. This exercise should deepen the Coalition's conversations by exploring the scope, type, and amount of change that is needed.

Instructions:

- Open the activity with high-level information about the case for change, the project community (who is in and who is out), the type of change (transformational), and other information that was generated in the previous activities.
- Invite participants to reflect in one of the following formats:
  - Speed-dating format:
    - One half of the Guiding Coalition forms an outer circle and the other half forms an inner circle. Each person from the inner circle should be partnered with one person from the outer circle. Participants discuss their answer to the prompt with their partner for 1 to 2 minutes and then switch partners (have one circle, inner or outer, rotate clockwise).
  - Fishbowl format:
    - One half of the Guiding Coalition forms an outer circle and the other half forms an inner circle. The participants in the inner circle discuss their answers to the prompt while the participants in the outer circle actively listen to the inner circle's discussion without contributing. The inner and outer circles switch after 10 minutes or until the discussion has reached a natural ending.
- Instruct members to begin processing the change characteristics using the following prompts:
  1. Type of change: developmental, transitional, and transformational? What does antiracism transformational change look like? How do we know if it is happening?
  2. Scope of the change: How big is this change? How many people are affected? Is this the right project community?

3. Amount of change: What is the amount of work that needs to be done?
- Reconvene as a larger group and invite participants to share final reflections and shared themes.

Activity 3d: Developing Vision, Values, and Guiding Principles

The next step is to focus on establishing a clear vision for your change and the values and core principles that will drive the Guiding Coalition's work. These are essential components of your change process roadmap and are crucial for success.

Future Traveler [12]

A vision can motivate and guide the actions of the Guiding Coalition and your project community, and it provides a basis for developing other aspects of your change process roadmap. Although individuals are motivated by different factors, a vision statement encourages people by presenting an achievable picture of what success looks like in the end. It can serve as a North Star, aligning efforts towards a common outcome. Your vision should provide realistic goals that are achievable and should be:
- understood and shared by members of the community;
- broad enough to include a variety of local perspectives;
- inspiring and uplifting to everyone involved in your effort; and
- easy to communicate.

Time expected to complete: 1.5 hours.

Target audience: Guiding Coalition members and other stakeholders in the project community. It is up to you to determine the right number of people involved in this exercise. If the target audience exceeds twenty people, we recommend facilitating multiple sessions.

Purpose of the activity: (1) To invite participants in the visioning process, describing vivid and detailed images of the future they want to cocreate; and (2) to achieve emotional resonance and assist you in supporting the change from a place of authenticity. If the change is already underway, this exercise may be used retrospectively to help you mitigate resistance and continue to move the Guiding Coalition through the change process.

Instructions:
- Set the context for participants (see sample script later).
- Instruct participants to close their eyes and relax.
- Suggest a series of images for them to imagine.

- Please allow adequate time after each of your suggested images for participants to reflect. Try to follow along with the imagery yourself so you can get a sense of how much time to leave.
- Read sample script.[12]
  - Context: *In order to get past the attitudes and real or perceived obstacles that sometimes make it hard for us to dream, it is helpful to take ourselves into the future and look backwards. We will be using a technique called guided imagery to assist us in doing this.*
  Please close your eyes.
  Take a few deep breaths and relax, settling your body into the chair.
  See a calendar, each page showing one date.
  See today's date. [state date]
  And now watch the pages turn, one by one... through to the end of this year... and into next year, month by month... and the next year, and the year after that... until you arrive at "x" years from today.
  It is "x" years in the future, and your vision has already been realized. All the things you are working for have come to pass. Your highest hopes have been achieved in just the ways you wanted.
  See the impact of your work in the world.
  See the impact of the Guiding Coalition's work.
  See the specific results that have been created.
  See the way the school has grown and developed.
  See what has rippled out into the world from your actions and from the Guiding Coalition's projects.
  See the lives of people being touched by your work. By our work.
- Allow for a few moments of silence and invite participants to open their eyes.
- Allow participants to share their future travel vision in breakout rooms or smaller groups. Each breakout room or small group should take notes using a shared document or online platform (e.g., Mural or Padlet) and begin constructing a vision statement they can share with the larger group. Return as a larger group to debrief.
- If you elicited examples of visions from your project community during the transformational kickoff communications, this debrief would be the time to share those examples with the Coalition.

- After the session, a smaller group should word-smith and finalize the vision.

Aligning Vision and Values

After you have developed a vision of what your future might look like, tap into your core values as an individual and an institution and find a way to anchor one or more of them to some aspect of the change. By aligning the institution's core values with your vision you can win the hearts and minds of the individuals needed to enact the change. Collectively, your vision and values will serve as a framework and tool to help your Guiding Coalition accomplish what it has set out to do.

Time expected to complete: 1 hour.

Target audience: Guiding Coalition members.

Purpose of the activity: To share personal and institutional values and connect them to the vision for change.

Instructions:

- With the list provided in Table 5.4, invite Guiding Coalition members to indicate their top five personal values. Add any that are missing that are meaningful to them. Now think about your values as a medical school or institution. Write down the top five institutional values.
- Ask Coalition members: "Looking at the identified values (personal and institutional), can you align one or more of the values to the vision? If so, how?"
- Debrief and ask the group to draft a set of three to four guiding principles, each no longer than one sentence. For each principle consider the following questions:

TABLE 5.4	**Values**	
Authenticity	Freedom	Kindness
Balance	Friendship	Knowledge
Commitment	Fun	Loyalty
Compassion	Generosity	Openness
Concern for others	Genuineness	Perseverance
Courage	Happiness	Personal growth
Creativity	Harmony	Respect for others
Education	Health	Responsibility
Empathy	Honesty	Security
Excellence	Humor	Serenity
Fairness	Integrity	Service to others
Faith	Intelligence	Success
Family	Joyfulness	

1. Will it draw people to the change?
2. Does it offer hope for a better future?
3. Will it inspire the project community to realize the vision through positive, effective action?
4. Does it provide a basis for developing the other aspects of your change process roadmap?
5. Does it describe what you will do and why you will do it?
6. Is it outcome-oriented?
7. Is it inclusive of the goals and people who may become involved in the change?

Activity 3e: Building an Infrastructure and Conditions to Support Change

Building an infrastructure and supports is an investment in the future.[1] The first step in creating an infrastructure that promotes long-term strategic change is identifying the conditions for success. Using this activity you can identify the infrastructure necessary to get to your future state.

Time expected to complete: 1 hour.

Target audience: Guiding Coalition members.

Purpose of the activity: To build a supportive infrastructure for change that will prepare, equip, and enable members of the Guiding Coalition to lead change.

Instructions:

During the activity the Coalition will identify systems, processes, and procedures that need to be in place or improved to ensure the change is successful.

- Introduce the importance of developing an infrastructure and support for the Coalition.
- Review these small group discussion questions/prompts with the Coalition:
  1. What type of infrastructure do we need to succeed? Think about the Guiding Coalition, spheres, roles, processes, structures, etc.
  2. How will we make decisions (governance structure) both in the Guiding Coalition and the spheres?
  3. How will we stay connected, communicate with each other, share resources, and troubleshoot?
  4. How will we ensure we are working collaboratively and not in silos?
  5. What barriers do we anticipate?
  6. What knowledge, skills, and resources are needed at this time?
  7. What systems, tools, and professional development opportunities are needed?

- Assign Guiding Coalition members to breakout rooms or small groups based on the spheres or functional areas. Ensure small groups are taking notes either on a shared document or other web-based platform (e.g., Jamboard, Slido, Padlet, etc.)
- Debrief as a large group and ensure that you have captured or collected all of the notes.
- Follow up with the Coalition on any items that need to be addressed. Share notes with the change strategy team in order to identify strategies that will support the Coalition over time.

Activity 3f: Communicating the Vision for Change, Strategy, and Process Across the School

The goal is to have a critical mass of people join in a concerted effort to participate in the change with clear purpose and resolve. All of the levels of the project community are access points for collective action. How do you establish that critical mass? There is no set formula, yet there are many options that have been identified by Anderson and Anderson:

- Widespread engagement through storytelling.
- Interactive dialogue that deepens people's understanding and builds their excitement.
- Planned experiences that impact people's mindsets and emotions.
- Opportunities for people to provide input on key change issues that demonstrably influence leadership thinking.
- Making the distinction overt between the limitations of old ways of operating and the value of new ways.
- Sharing responsibilities for critical action and authority with all levels of the institution.

Time expected to complete: 1 hour.

Target audience: Guiding Coalition members.

Purpose of the activity: To create collective intention in order to produce transformational results.

Instructions:

- Start by illustrating the importance of communicating the vision effectively as a key quality during periods of change. Keep the message simple by telling stories to demonstrate benefits; remain authentic and approachable; and help members of the project community come to their own understanding in a manner that is consistent with the change initiative's vision of the future. By doing this you will better engage members of the project community and motivate them to become integral players in the change.
- Assign Guiding Coalition members to breakout rooms or small groups based on the spheres or functional areas. Ensure small groups are taking notes.
- Instruct each group to consider their stakeholders. In the small breakout groups, generate a communication strategy to ensure that the stakeholder group will be able to answer the following key questions (See Worksheet 5.5: Communication Strategy):
  1. What is the vision?
  2. What is my role in achieving this vision?
  3. What are the obstacles preventing me from contributing to the vision?
  4. Can I explain the vision and its importance to others?
  5. What is the process (roadmap) for getting us to the vision?
- When developing the communications strategy, consider:
  - Storytelling
  - Interactive dialogue that deepens stakeholders' understanding and builds their excitement
  - Planned experiences that impact stakeholders' mindsets and emotions
  - Opportunities for people to provide input
  - Making the distinction overt between the limitations of old ways of operating and the value of new ways
  - Sharing responsibilities for critical action and authority
- Debrief sphere communication strategies with the large group. Each sphere should agree on a timeline for rolling out the communication strategy. Ideally, all spheres will be communicating the vision and the roadmap to each of their stakeholder groups.
- Follow up with each sphere and troubleshoot any issues.

Our Experience: Early Year of the Guiding Coalition

One of the Guiding Coalition's earliest and most important tasks was to decide whether we would be tackling all forms of bias, just racism, or bias with a particular focus on racism. We could not in good conscience ignore the many other forms of oppression perpetuated in academic medicine. At the same time, taking on all forms of bias risked diluting the impact we could have on any one area of concern. Despite not reaching full agreement, we decided to focus on racism first, recognizing that it was the most deeply rooted, profoundly impactful of all the biases, and was threaded through the practice of medicine, biomedical research, and medical education.

The decision to focus on racism led to our vision statement: To become a health system and health professions school with the most diverse workforce, providing health care and education that is free of racism and bias. The Guiding Coalition was intentionally bold and aspirational in crafting the vision, recognizing that there was no known end point in achieving this desired state. Thus the values of the Guiding Coalition had to be anchored in disrupting some existing norms and characteristics by naming them when they occurred, and role modeling the antidotes to these characteristics in our work with one another and with our stakeholders.

2023 marks 5 years since the launch of the Racism and Bias Initiative (RBI) and formation of our Guiding Coalition. Since its inception, every activity has been linked to communicating our vision for change, our strategy, and the process for change. We continue to use multiple traditional platforms (newsletters, email updates, blog posts) to engage others in this work. We also use the activities of the RBI to achieve this goal. For example, in our Chats of Change series (see Chapter 9 for details), we share the history and vision of our journey at the start of every chat dialogue. The open-access portfolio of change targets developed by our Guiding Coalition is another way of communicating our vision, strategy, and change process with all members of our project community.

REFERENCES

1. Anderson LA, Anderson D. *The Change Leader's Roadmap: How to Navigate Your Organization's Transformation.* Vol. 384. Hoboken, NJ: John Wiley & Sons; 2010.
2. Hiatt J. *ADKAR: A Model for Change in Business, Government and Our Community.* Loveland, CO: Prosci Research; 2006. https://copdei.extension.org/wp-content/uploads/2019/06/Organizational-Climate-and-Culture-Review.pdf.
3. Schneider B, Ehrhart MG, Macey WH. Organizational climate and culture. *Annu Rev Psychol.* 2013;64:361-388. doi:10.1146/annurev-psych-113011-143809.
4. Kotter JP. *Accelerate! Harvard Business Review.* 2015. https://hbr.org/2012/11/accelerate.
5. Farhang L, Gould S. *Racial Justice and Power-Sharing: The Heart of Leading Systems Change.* Oregon Health Authority; 2021. https://www.oregon.gov/oha/OHPB/MtgDocs/1.2%20Systems%20Change%20Article.pdf.
6. Bates K, Parker CS, Ogden C. *Power Dynamics: The Hidden Element to Effective Meetings.* Interaction Institute for Social Change; 2018. https://interactioninstitute.org/power-dynamics-the-hidden-element-to-effective-meetings/.
7. Harvard University. *Calling In and Calling Out Guide.* https://edib.harvard.edu/files/dib/files/calling_in_and_calling_out_guide_v4.pdf?m=1625683246.
8. Bono DE. *New Think: The Use of Lateral Thinking in the Generation of New Ideas.* New York, NY: Basic Books; 1967.
9. CRR Global. *About ORSC.* 2022. https://crrglobal.com/about/orsc/.
10. Teamcatapult. *Creating Safe Space for Organizational Transformation.* 2013. https://www.top-network.org/assets/images/monthlyfeatures/2013June/participant%20workbook%20final.pdf.
11. He Y, Hutson BL, Bloom JL. Appreciative Team Building in Learning Organizations. Scholarly inquiry in academic advising: NACADA Monograph Series M. 2010;20:133-141.
12. Gass R. *Future Travel Exercise.* Art of Transformation Consulting; 2013. https://atctools.org/toolkit_tool/future-travel-exercise/.

6

Phase 4: Engaging and Enabling Your Institution for Change

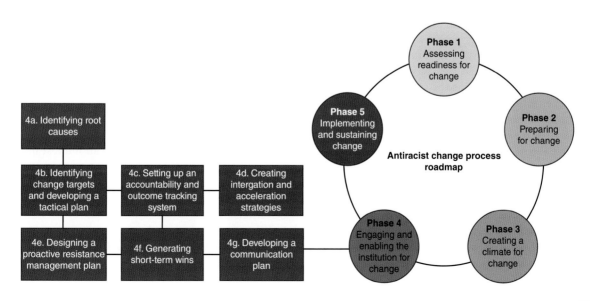

MOVING DEEPER INTO MIDSTREAM CHANGE

The goal of phase 4 is to set up the conditions that will engage and enable your institution for change. During this phase the Guiding Coalition will broaden its reach by actively engaging members of the project community, giving them the capability and confidence to know what is changing and the process for getting there.

It is no secret that highly engaged people improve performance in organizations. When it comes to transformational change, they can also make the transition from the current state to the future state more quickly and effectively. When introducing change, especially change related to dismantling racism, it is vitally important to keep engagement high, ensuring all individuals know enough about the change so that they can embrace the change and encourage it in all the constituents with whom they interact.[1]

Although American society has been in the midst of a racial reckoning where it is no longer acceptable to ignore racist structures, practices, policies, and behaviors, you will likely also experience and witness the anger, resentment, and fear that often follows discussions of racism and explorations of antiracism.[2] Engaging and enabling your project community to move towards antiracist transformation becomes even more challenging when you are confronted with "system-justifying beliefs that raise questions about deservingness, legitimize the status quo, and therefore defend inaction."[3] It is important to expect this type of resistance, especially during phase 4, and to devote the time needed to tend to the human component of change.[2]

This chapter will outline the seven steps for engaging and enabling people within your project community or institution for change. We will provide detailed instructions on how to execute each of the seven steps (we call them "activities"), and where applicable we will share our experience as it relates to the change process. First, we invite your Guiding Coalition to consider employing the following antiracist practices: naming the discomfort, labeling emotions and bringing them out into the open.

Antiracist practices. While completing the seven activities, consider the following antiracist practice.

NAME THE DISCOMFORT: LABELING EMOTIONS AND BRINGING THEM OUT INTO THE OPEN

The emotional work of antiracism requires that we gain more awareness of the mindset that is deeply embedded in our culture. When completing the seven steps for engaging and enabling your project community, try to identify how these cultural characteristics are showing up. Drawing from the work of Tema Okun, we invite you to consider how the *right to comfort* and *fear of open conflict* manifest in the Guiding Coalition and members of your project community.[4] For example, when someone raises an issue that causes discomfort, what is the response? Is the response to blame the person for raising the issue rather than examining what is actually causing the problem? Is there even space or time dedicated to discussing the issue itself? Is there an emphasis on being polite and an assumption that raising difficult issues is impolite, rude, or out of line? Who is setting the rules for how ideas, information or differences of opinion need to be shared in order to be heard (for example, requiring that people "calm down" if they are angry)? Is there a culture of punishing people either overtly or subtly for speaking out about their truth and/or experience? In what ways are people labeling emotion either explicitly or implicitly as irrational, antiintellectual, or inferior, thereby failing to recognize the importance of emotional intelligence?

Deeply entrenched social and cultural norms create and sustain the structures that privilege or oppress others, and are aligned with certain emotional attachments.[2,5] Challenging those norms means changing our emotional relationship to them. Given that there are people who are privileged by these norms, they tend not to be given up easily. If our goal is transformation, our approach cannot afford to ignore how to access the deep emotional knowledge experienced by people who are most likely to resist change. As an individual, you can personally take an interest in your own emotional intelligence when you are activated or experience discomfort related to race, racism, and antiracism. Consider the following Self-Reflection Questions:

1. When you are activated, who do you become? How do you behave? What sensations, emotions, and thoughts do you notice?

2. What patterns of soothing and regulation do you notice? How do you move away from discomfort? What are your escape routes?
3. What can you do to build stamina for leaning into discomfort?
4. Who are the people with whom you can process?

As a Coalition, you can set antiracist group norms that encourage full participation and strive to decenter expectations of "comfort." You can use these norms in your Guiding Coalition meetings and when convening your project community. This list of norms is not exhaustive or static.[6]

- *Recognize.* We recognize that we must strive to overcome historical and divisive biases, such as racism and sexism, in our society.
- *Acknowledge.* We acknowledge that we are all systematically taught misinformation about our own group(s) and about members of other groups.
- *No blame.* We agree not to blame ourselves or others for the misinformation we have learned, but to accept responsibility for not repeating misinformation after we have learned otherwise.
- *Respect.* We agree to treat other participants' reflections and questions with respect. We acknowledge that we may be at different stages of learning on any given topic. However, this does not mean we should ignore problematic statements.
- *Individual experience.* We agree that no one should be required or expected to speak for their whole race or social identity group.
- *Share the air.* Share responsibility for including all voices in the discussion. If you have a tendency to dominate discussions, take a step back and help the group invite others to speak. If you tend to stay quiet, challenge yourself to share ideas so others can learn from you. If you are exceedingly quiet, expect that the facilitator may call on you in meetings to participate.
- *Not experts.* The facilitators are not experts. They are here to help facilitate the process. They and everyone in the group are here to learn. We also recognize that everyone has an opinion. Opinions, however, are not the same as informed knowledge backed up by research. Depending on the topic and context, both are valid to share, but it is important to know the difference. To engage in deep learning, we will want to lean more toward informed knowledge and gain practice reflecting and speaking thoughtfully about difficult topics.
- *Ask for help.* It is okay not to know. Keep in mind that we are all still learning and are bound to make mistakes when approaching a complex task or exploring new ideas. Be open to changing your mind, and make space for others to do so as well.

SEVEN STEPS FOR ENGAGING AND ENABLING YOUR INSTITUTION FOR CHANGE

These steps do not need to be completed in order, although we have scaffolded these activities to build on one another. We recommend that you treat these steps as iterative and continue to update or refine them as new information becomes available. It is important to consider who needs to inform each of the steps and what voices and perspectives should be included.

Identifying Root Causes

The first step involves identifying root causes with stakeholders from your project community. This is done by using a systems thinking tool called the *iceberg model* that will help you gain perspective on the whole system before identifying where to intervene and what should change.

Identifying Change Targets and Developing a Tactical Plan

The second step focuses on determining what needs to change and creating a tactical plan.

The Guiding Coalition will use the iceberg model results to identify change targets or areas of intervention that could lead to systemic transformation, and create a tactical plan for that transformation.

Establishing a Change Target Outcome Tracking System

The third step involves using Results-Based Accountability (RBA) to monitor and track outcomes and outputs related to the quantity (how much was done), quality (how well it was done), and impact (if anyone is better off) of the change targets.

Creating Integration and Acceleration Strategies

The fourth step starts by creating an integration strategy that ensures the change targets are aligned and not competing for resources, overlapping in scope, overtaxing capacity, sending mixed messages, or duplicating efforts. The Guiding Coalition will then consider conditions that slow down change, and brainstorm strategies to resolve those conditions or prevent them from happening in the first place.

Designing a Proactive Resistance Management Plan

The fifth step focuses on proactive resistance management that will address anticipated or identified sources of resistance.

Generating Short-term Wins

The sixth step focuses on intentionally generating short-term wins in order to keep the project community engaged and to prevent loss of momentum.

Developing a Communication Plan and Closing the Loop

The seventh step circles back to the sponsor and project community. The Guiding Coalition will develop a communication plan to share the change targets, as well as the process for achieving the antiracist vision.

PHASE 4 ACTIVITIES AND INSTRUCTIONS

Activity 4a: Identifying Root Causes

You cannot identify where and what should change within a system without first understanding the system itself. The application of a systems thinking tool called the iceberg model allows us to look at a system through different lenses and provides a way to talk about the experiences we each have of what is happening in the system. It forces us to expand our horizons and not limit ourselves to looking at just a single event, but to step back and identify the patterns that that event is part of, the structures that might be contributing to those patterns, the thinking that is sustaining those structures, and the cultural and institutional values that underpin and make up our worldview.

Time expected to complete: 1.5 hours; we recommend facilitating a series of meetings with the target audience to maximize engagement and ensure a diversity of perspectives.

Target audience: Members or representatives of your entire project community.

Purpose of the activity: To uncover root causes by looking at hidden levels within the system that are not immediately obvious.

Instructions Fig. 6.1[7]:

- Introduce the concept of the iceberg using the following talking points and diagram:
  - When we look at an iceberg, typically a very small portion of it is visible above the water line. The vast majority is submerged. We are going to pay attention to what is visible, as well as explore what might be happening beneath the surface.
    - *Events.* Above the water line are the events—they are the "what happened," the newspaper headlines, the "what we saw"—and they often appear to be discreet episodes.
    - *Patterns of events.* Moving just below the waterline are patterns of events. If you look at events over some period of time you will start to notice patterns or trends. Patterns answer the questions, "what has been happening" or "what is changing?" If you expand the time period broadly enough, eventually all events will show up as part of a pattern. It is important to be careful here: only the events are real data; patterns require some interpretation of the data. Sometimes one can be fooled into believing that there is a pattern when none exists. It is important to get group agreement as to whether a pattern is really evident.
    - *Underlying structures.* Below the patterns of events are the underlying structures that are causing those patterns of events to occur. Structures are the "rules of the game." They can be written or unwritten; they can be physical and visible or invisible. They are norms, policies, guidelines, power structures, distribution of resources, cultural rules, or informal ways of working that have been tacitly or explicitly institutionalized. They answer the question "How did this pattern emerge?"
    - *Mental models.* Below the structures are the mental models. These define the thinking that creates the structures that then manifest themselves in the patterns of events. Mental models are people's deeply held assumptions and beliefs, whether conscious ("I know I think like this") or unconscious ("I have always thought this way and do not

The iceberg
Tool for guiding systemic thinking

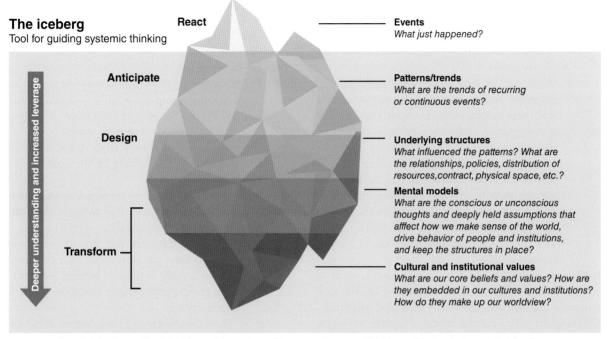

Fig. 6.1 Iceberg Model (Adapted from Reos Partners. *Systems Thinking with the Iceberg Module.* Reos Partners; 2015. https://reospartners.com/publications/systems-thinking-with-the-iceberg-module/.[7])

even question it, the idea is so core to my being"), that drive behavior.

- *Cultural and institutional values.* Lastly, below the mental models are cultural and institutional values: the core beliefs embedded in our institutions(s) that make up our worldview. These shape our mental models and are seldom brought to the surface to be seen, named, examined, or challenged. Here we encourage you to consider some typical culture characteristics.[4]
- Use an example to walk the group through the thinking process. (Use your own or the following one.)
  - First we want to identify a critical event that we feel reveals something important about the system we are trying to understand. Remember that an event is observable and is the "what happened."
  - Then we want to describe the event in some detail. For example: last Tuesday we

had a meeting at 3 p.m. and Mille arrived 20 minutes late. Write this fact down on a large (4" × 6") Post-it and stick it on the "events" part of the iceberg. You can also use web-based platforms like Mural to virtually place the Post-it on the "events" part of the iceberg.

- Now we want to identify some of the patterns that this event may be part of. For example, maybe one person said that Mille is always late.
- One of the other people in the group said that that was not true; it was just that Mille was late this time. (For this step, we need to agree as a group that the pattern is plausible.)
- But there are lots of times that other people in this group are late coming to the meetings. (On a smaller Post-it write, "Many people are late to the meetings," and stick it on the "pattern" part of the iceberg.)
- What other patterns might Mille's lateness be part of? More people are late when it is raining.

(Write that on another small Post-it and stick it on the iceberg.) We have observed that more people are late when the meeting is at 3 p.m. as opposed to 4 p.m. (Write down and post that observation.)

- What sort of structures might explain these patterns? Traffic close to rush hour is terrible and there is little public transportation, so the transportation system is a problem. Everyone is forced to work the same business hours, so office policies are problematic. Often there is no agenda to the meeting so it is unclear why we are meeting. (Write each structure on a Post-it note and post the notes in the "structure" area of the iceberg.)
- Tell the group that you will look at mental models shortly.

Facilitator note: The reason we use Post-it notes is that we may want to move things around. We may decide that something initially identified as a structure is actually a mental model, a pattern may be a structure, etc. The idea is that we are making our thinking about this situation visible. Although it is helpful to get most of the patterns in the "pattern" category on the iceberg and the structures in the "structure" category, if the group cannot agree it is fine if items end up on the iceberg wherever folks are most comfortable.

- Also, please note that some people consider mental models to be structures. We find it useful to tease these categories apart and make the thinking explicit.
- **Talking points:**
  - Note that there is not just *one* pattern, structure, or mental model at play. There can be many. How you see things often depends on your vantage point within the system.
  - The core idea here is that the "whole is visible in the parts." The events are a reflection of larger patterns and structures. By looking at one event and how it came to pass, we will be able to perceive the larger whole.
  - The lower we go in the iceberg, the more leverage we have for transforming the system. Changing structures and influencing mental models has a broader, more far-reaching effect than reacting in the moment and fighting fires.

- Many times, it does not really matter which critical event we start with. We often end up identifying the same mental models and structures.
- **Do the exercise.**
  - *Option 1*
    - Ask the group to identify a critical event: What is a "newspaper headline" regarding the issue we are trying to address?
    - Write this event on a large Post-it note and stick it on the iceberg in the area labeled "Events."
    - Then ask the group to take a longer view: What are some of the patterns that this event might be part of?
    - Write the patterns that are identified on Post-its (one per note) and stick the notes on the iceberg in the area labeled "Patterns." The group needs to agree that these patterns are accurate.
    - Then ask the group to dig deeper: What are some of the structures that might be causing these patterns to occur? What are the relationships, policies, distribution of resources, job roles/responsibilities, physical space, etc.?
    - Write the structures that are identified on Post-its and stick them on the iceberg in the area labeled "Structures."

Facilitator note: Sometimes the group may come up with a pattern when talking about events, or a structure when talking about patterns or mental models. Feel free to challenge the group by asking, is this really a pattern or is it a structure? You can also ask people to look over the whole diagram at the end and make any adjustments by moving the Post-its around.

- *Option 2*
  - Break the group into smaller teams of about four to five people. Ask them to work using the previous process. Give each team a sheet of newsprint with the iceberg and events/patterns/structures/mental models listed on it and the two types of Post-its.
  - As the teams work, the facilitator walks around to coach and support them. Sometimes a team can get stuck on choosing the "right" event.

The teams need to choose an event that they observed in enough detail to tell a short story about it. They might get stuck on whether something is a pattern or a structure; in this case, have them put the Post-it on the line between the two. Do not let people get caught up in debate, unless it is around whether something actually has happened or whether the pattern is valid.

- **When the teams are finished, have them present their icebergs to each other.**
- **Debrief the icebergs.** What do we notice about them? What structures appear on more than one iceberg? What are the similarities? What are the outliers?
- **Make the mental models explicit.**
  - Go back to our previous example: Let us identify the mental models that created these structures. For instance, we do not trust our employees to work flexible hours. Public transportation is not worth the investment. The only way we will get anything done is if we are in the office during the same hours. (Write each mental model on a Post-it and stick the Post-it notes on the "mental model" area of the iceberg.)
  - In the same teams, look at the events, patterns, and structures that were identified and uncover the mental models that the group feels are at play in the system behind their iceberg picture.
    - What is the thinking that is creating the structures that are causing the events and patterns to occur?
    - What are the conscious and unconscious thoughts and deeply held assumptions that affect how we make sense of the world, drive the behavior of people and institutions, and keep the structures in place?
  - The iceberg model—and the conversation about mental models that it engenders—is a powerful way for members of a group to better understand the system within which they are working, as well as their own connection to the circumstances.
  - Try to give time to check in with participants and debrief about what is coming up for them when making these mental models explicit.

- **Uncover the cultural and institutional values that influence the mental models.**[8]
  - Lastly, ask Guiding Coalition members to consider the institution's core beliefs and values.
    - How are they embedded in our culture and institutions?
    - How do they make up our worldview and influence our mental models?
  - Introduce White supremacy culture characteristics and talk about how or whether they influence our values and mental models.[4]

Our Experience: Using the Iceberg Model to Identify the Root Causes in Our Institution

In the early stages of our Guiding Coalition we made a conscious effort not to be reactive by jumping to identify what needed to change. From a systems perspective, we knew we needed to engage more people across our institution to better understand how racism and bias were manifesting in all of the functional areas of our medical education program (our project community). As a result, each of the six Guiding Coalition spheres (admissions, curricular affairs, student affairs, students, clinical, and 'student resources'—housing, security, bursars office, etc.) facilitated a series of iceberg model sessions with their stakeholder groups. Each of the spheres identified an event that impacted its functional area. For example, the clinical sphere identified an event related to inequity in clerkship evaluations. Over the course of a few months, the data that was captured in the iceberg sessions was shared with staff, students, and faculty. Investing this time in listening to people ensured that we would make strategic decisions about the change that were broader than our narrow perspective. Our Guiding Coalition was then able to identify what needed to change in order to address the root causes, not just fix or react to events at the tip of the iceberg. This approach also created an opportunity for people across our medical school to contribute to the change on a larger scale and start to build meaningful buy-in. For some, especially frontline staff, this was the first time that they had been involved in the process of change.

Activity 4b: Identifying Change Targets and Developing a Tactical Plan

Once members of your project community have looked at the system through different lenses using the iceberg model, the Guiding Coalition can conduct a ZIP (zoom in; *i*nnovation opportunity; *p*roblem areas) analysis to identify at least one change target: an incremental desired outcome that strategically leads towards the coalition's vision.[9] The ZIP analysis provides a framework for the Guiding Coalition to identify potential areas for intervention and innovation that can be used as leverage points for impacting the system. These key points, or levers of change, should be informed by the iceberg model's conclusions. Leverage points are places in the system where, as systems theorist Donella Meadows posits, "a small shift in one thing can produce big changes in everything."[10] These leverage points create a cascading effect to produce big changes, just as removing a single load-bearing wall can bring down an entire house. While identifying these levers, we recommend considering the conditions that hold the problem in place.[11]

Once you have identified these leverage points, the next step is to turn them into change targets. From there the Guiding Coalition will be able to develop a tactical plan outlining the steps needed to achieve the change targets.

Time expected to complete: 3 hours; we recommend scheduling a series of meetings.

Target audience: Guiding Coalition members.

Purpose of the activity: To conduct a ZIP analysis to develop change targets or potential areas for intervention and innovation, and a tactical plan.

Instructions:

- *Content framing.* Define levers of change and introduce the six conditions of systems change:
  - *Levers of change.* Points of entry or leverage where intervention could lead to systemic transformation.[10] These levers are places where a small shift in one thing can produce big changes in everything. Similar to a domino effect, one action can cause a cascading effect over time. Sometimes this effect can surprise us later, when we least expect it (Fig. 6.2).
  - *The six conditions of systems change.* Interdependent conditions that often play significant roles in holding environmental or social problems in place.[11] In Fig. 6.3 you will see that these conditions exist in varying degrees of visibility (explicit, semiexplicit, and implicit) within a particular system. When identifying levers, consider where you might intervene to address the six conditions that are holding the root causes in place. Shifts in these six conditions are more likely to be

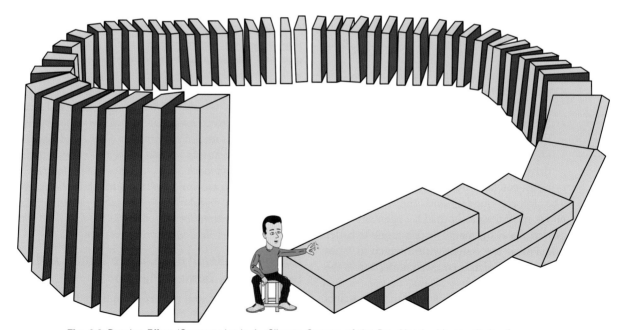

Fig. 6.2 Domino Effect (Courtesy Levin A. *Climate Cartoon of the Day.* Used with permission from www. CartoonStock.com.[12])

Six conditions of systems change

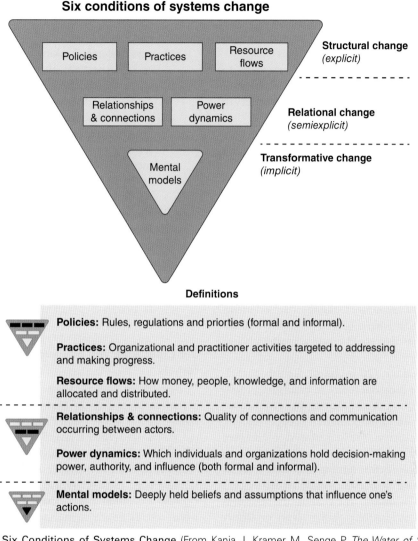

Structural change
(explicit)

Relational change
(semiexplicit)

Transformative change
(implicit)

Definitions

Policies: Rules, regulations and priorties (formal and informal).

Practices: Organizational and practitioner activities targeted to addressing and making progress.

Resource flows: How money, people, knowledge, and information are allocated and distributed.

Relationships & connections: Quality of connections and communication occurring between actors.

Power dynamics: Which individuals and organizations hold decision-making power, authority, and influence (both formal and informal).

Mental models: Deeply held beliefs and assumptions that influence one's actions.

Fig. 6.3 Six Conditions of Systems Change (From Kania J, Kramer M, Senge P. *The Water of Systems Change.* FSG Reimagining Social Change; 2018. https://philea.issuelab.org/resources/30855/30855.pdf.[11])

sustained when targeting your change on all three levels.[11]

- Conduct a ZIP analysis to identify levers of change. Note: this step should consider the information that was captured during the iceberg exercise (Activity 4a: Identifying Root Causes).

ZIP analysis focuses on the following:

- *Zoom in.* What should we focus on? What should we magnify and explore further? What needs additional research or investigation?

Based on the idea of entry or leverage points, where might we start?

- *Innovation opportunity.* At this time, are there any innovation opportunities that we should consider? What ways can we intervene to improve the system and address racism and bias? To what extent have your, or our, actions contributed to the conditions holding the problem in place? To what extent have actions you/we have witnessed contributed to holding the problem in place? Where do we see levers for change that could cause a great impact from a small change? When identifying the innovation opportunities consider working on all levels to address the six conditions of systems change.

- *Problem areas.* What are the tricky areas to navigate, pain points or potential roadblocks? What unforeseen areas could create barriers to enacting these levers or opportunities?

We recommend conducting the analysis in a series of small group breakouts and large group debrief sessions.

- **Z breakout (20 minutes):** Split the larger group into groups of five to six people and instruct each small group to focus on the "Z." Utilize the information gained from the iceberg model and answer the questions proposed earlier.
- **Debrief (10 minutes):** After the small group breakout, bring the groups back together to debrief as a whole. Reinforce systems thinking where necessary and encourage Guiding Coalition members to consider what might be magnified and explored further that could create a greater change impact.
- **I and P breakout (20 minutes):** Return participants to their breakout rooms to brainstorm innovation opportunities and identify any problem areas. When brainstorming innovation opportunities, encourage participants to look inward at their own behaviors and how they contribute to holding the problem in place before turning externally. Instruct them to answer the questions outlined earlier.
- **Debrief (20 minutes):** The goal of this session is to end with at least one *change target* or clearly defined area where there is a need for change. Encourage participants to mold their innovation opportunities or levers for change into a sentence that is outcome-based and people-dependent.
  - Based on the identified levers, what incremental end result(s) or outcome(s) do we want to achieve that will lead us towards our vision? Change targets should focus on outcomes or results that can be achieved in 1 to 2 years. We recommend having the Guiding Coalition spheres create change target(s) related to their functional areas or topics of focus. Weigh the pros and cons of the number of change targets to take on. Do not assume that more change targets will produce bigger or greater change.

This is the time to be strategic and transform the reactive "fix it" approach that normally keeps us busy but not productive. Instead, we should harness systems thinking and the diverse voices and perspectives that have been generated. Often the change targets begin to emerge organically as the Guiding Coalition engages in dialogue about the levers of change while using the iceberg model results. During the dialogue, it might be helpful to visibly take notes so that members of the Guiding Coalition can generate agreement or edit where they see fit.

- An example of a change target:

Enhance growth in personal awareness, antiracist knowledge, and skills among course and clerkship directors who are frontline voices to students and faculty. As you can see there is a specific outcome (increase in personal awareness and antiracist knowledge and skills) that is people-dependent (course and clerkship directors).

Our Experience: RBI Guiding Coalition 2022 Change Targets

Developing Tactical Plan. *In 2022 our Guiding Coalition committed to 24 change targets.*[13] *Even though change targets might change each year, they align us to our vision—to become a health system and health profession school with the most diverse workforce, providing health care, education, and research that are free of racism and bias.* Table 6.1 *provides a sampling of our 2022 Guiding Coalition's change targets by sphere, including which conditions of system change they aimed to target.*

- Introduce the *Graphic Gameplan* to create a tactical plan for each change target. We recommend using the Graphic Gameplan that was created by The Grove Consultants International.[14] The Graphic Gameplan is a graphic organizer that allows groups to visualize their target(s) and the stages and tasks needed to get there, along with the success factors and the challenges that will be faced along the way. By using this graphic organizer the Guiding Coalition can turn its plans and words into action.
- Introduce the Graphic Gameplan to the Guiding Coalition. Depending on the design of your Guiding Coalition, every sphere can work on its own Graphic Gameplan for each of its change targets.

TABLE 6.1 **Sample of 2022 Change Targets**		
Racism and Bias Initiative Guiding Coalition Sphere	**Change Target Statement**	**Condition of System Change**
Admissions	Increase the capacity of the Admissions Committee to continually engage in admissions work through an equity lens.	Structural
Curricular affairs	Pilot a standardized patient session on navigating patients or colleagues who manifest racist behaviors during clinical encounters, both as a student who is under-represented in medicine and as an ally.	Structural
Resources	Create a process whereby medical education staff can share resources for practicing antiracism as a business practice.	Structural
Student affairs	Increase the capacity of faculty advisors to coach students through difficult situations and commit to an ongoing practice of applying appreciative advising strategies.	Structural
Students	Increase visibility of and provide opportunities for collaboration with and among student groups in order to reduce silos among stakeholder groups involved in antiracism work.	Relational
Clinical environment	Enhance the comfort of the Sinai community to discuss issues related to racism in clinical practice, and their familiarity with mechanisms for reporting racism and bias.	Transformative
School wide	Enhance capacity among senior medical education leaders to integrate a trauma-informed approach when addressing racism and bias and other forms of oppression in their work and learning environments.	Transformative

Alternatively, the entire Guiding Coalition can create one master Graphic Gameplan.

- Are your objectives process- or outcome-oriented?
  - Process objectives describe the activities or strategies that will be used as part of achieving your change targets. Process objectives, by their nature, are usually short term.
    - Example: By (month/year), (X%) of faculty will be contacted (via communications and engagement opportunities) within (time period) to build buy-in and awareness of how racism is impacting our learning environment and begin to build the case for why faculty development is needed.
  - Outcome objectives specify the intended effect of the change target or end result. The outcome objectives focus on what your project community will know or be able to do as a result of the change target.
    - Example: By (month/year), faculty who attended (x training sessions) will demonstrate an increase in antiracist practices during their lectures and small group sessions.

- In the area labeled, *Other Objectives*, write down any other objectives.
- In the area labeled *Stages/Tasks* (above the large arrow), write down the major stages. Each stage should align with one column within the large arrow. Inside of the large arrow, write down the individual tasks that must be completed for each stage in the corresponding column.
- In the area labeled *Challenges*, write down the challenges the Guiding Coalition and/or sphere will face along the way.
- In the area labeled *SUCCESS FACTORS*, write down the success factors for the project.

Once completed, you can transfer the Post-it note content to Worksheet 6.1 Graphic Gameplan Notes Template.

Our Experience: Tactical Plan

Initially the graphic organizer was a helpful tool that helped us engage our Guiding Coalition in a collaborative planning process. Prior to this initiative, leaders or managers would develop a plan and roll it out through a traditional top-down mechanism. In the Guiding Coalition we did not want to rely on this practice because we knew it would not produce the full-thickness engagement and collaboration needed for transformation. The graphic organizer disrupted the status quo. When it was first introduced there were a lot of questions about how it worked and concerns about getting it right. At some point, we just had to trust the experience and lean into it. After we were done developing the tactical plan, Coalition members commented positively on how productive they were and on the end result. In hindsight, the graphic organizer allowed us to plan as a team and provided a visual aid for us to see how the intricate parts related to the overarching plan. The organizer served as a guide that kept us on track and focused.

Activity 4c: Setting Up an Accountability and Outcome Tracking System

Now that each change target has a corresponding tactical plan, you are ready to establish a means of tracking your change target outcomes over time. We recommend using RBA to create a plan for collecting data and monitoring outcomes. RBA is a disciplined way of thinking about and solving entrenched and complex social problems. Developed by Mark Friedman and described in his book *Trying Hard is Not Good Enough*,[15] RBA is used in communities and organizations to shift from talking about problems to taking action and solving problems. The benefits of employing RBA make it an ideal framework for transformational change and ensure your change targets are leading towards tangible outcomes, not just checking off boxes. RBA is a simple, common-sense process that everyone can understand. It builds collaboration and consensus and uses data and transparency to ensure accountability. On the most basic level, RBA will allow the Guiding Coalition to monitor and track how much it does, how well it is doing, and if anyone in the project community is better off.
Time expected to complete: 1.5 hours.
Target audience: Guiding Coalition members.
Purpose of the activity: To set up an RBA framework for tracking change target outcomes over time.
Instructions:
- Introduce RBA to the Guiding Coalition.
- Instruct each Guiding Coalition sphere to complete each quadrant of the RBA worksheet by answering the questions in the box (Worksheet 6.2).
- Once complete, the spheres should share their RBA plan with the Guiding Coalition and those in the project community.

- The change strategy team can create a master spreadsheet (Excel or Smartsheet) so each sphere can track and share their data internally with the Guiding Coalition.
- We recommend that the Guiding Coalition report out on its RBA data on a yearly basis. The data can be used for future planning sessions and for communications with the project community.

Our Experience: Results-Based Accountability (RBA) – Is Anyone Better Off? How do You Know?

The RBA framework is perhaps the most challenging step of the tactical plan. After 2 years of implementing change we needed a standardized way of monitoring our impact over time. We came across RBA as a methodology and decided to implement it into our planning process.

Despite the clear guidance on how to complete the RBA, it was challenging because it forced us to change the way in which we thought about our change efforts. Determining the accountability measures for each change target required us to think about our outcomes and end results first, then determine our efforts (quantity and quality) and evidence of effect or impact. This was not easy for many of our Coalition members because we had never held ourselves accountable in this way. Since this type of accountability was not coming from the top down, it meant that we were holding each other accountable. We continue to question if we are capturing the right data to determine if anyone is better off based on our efforts. This disciplined way of thinking was a new practice for us and required intention and persistence.

Activity 4d: Creating Integration and Acceleration Strategies

The next step ensures that the Guiding Coalition spheres are integrating efforts and accelerating change. Guiding Coalition members will first identify an integration strategy to ensure their change targets, tactical plans, and tracking systems are aligned and not competing for resources, overlapping in scope, overtaxing capacity, sending mixed messages, or duplicating efforts. Once the integration strategy is identified, the Guiding Coalition will consider conditions that slow down change and brainstorm strategies to resolve those conditions or prevent them from happening in the first place.
Time expected to complete: 1 hour.
Target audience: Guiding Coalition members.

Purpose of the activity: To identify integration and acceleration strategies that will strengthen the Guiding Coalition's efforts.

Instructions:

- Using the following questions, engage in a large or small group discussion about integration:
  - Are any of the change targets, tactical plans, and tracking systems competing for resources, overlapping in scope, overtaxing capacity, sending mixed messages, or duplicating efforts? If so, what changes can be made?
  - Are there any efforts that should be aligned or coordinated?
  - Are there new ways of working together that could help integrate efforts and break down silos?
  - What structures can be put into place to monitor integration of efforts?
- Engage in a large or small group discussion about acceleration using the following discussion questions[1]:
  - What causes change to slow down? Organize the answers into themes. For each theme, discuss how you might respond to or proactively plan for the slowdown.
  - How will you set up our change efforts to ensure optimal speed without cutting corners?
  - How will you ensure that strategies are designed to minimize negative impacts on the people who are involved in the change? How can you implement antiracist practices?
- Record answers and share them with the Guiding Coalition. Revisit when necessary. You can also add strategies generated from this session to the Graphic Gameplan Notes Template.

Our Experience: Integration

Integration has always been a challenge because of the siloed nature of our medical school and the design of our Guiding Coalition. In the beginning we created spheres that were representative of all the functional areas of the school. The great benefit of this design was that working within each sphere/functional area allowed us to streamline and standardize our approach. On the other hand, this approach also reinforced working within existing silos.

We were not intentional about prioritizing integration and acceleration strategies when we first began and had to contend with some negative downstream consequences of not planning for integration. We subsequently developed change targets with associated integration strategies to intentionally disrupt our silos and promote more broad-based action across our functional areas.

Activity 4e: Designing a Proactive Resistance Management Plan

Resistance to change should be expected, especially when embarking on a journey towards antiracism. Instead of being surprised when it emerges, the Guiding Coalition and others engaging and enabling your institution or project community for change can proactively anticipate and identify sources of resistance.

Prosci uses the word "resistance" to describe the physiological and psychological responses to change that manifest in specific behaviors.[16] Resistance can occur throughout the various states of change (e.g., leaving the current state, going through the transition state, arriving in the future state). The goal is to be able to recognize and determine the links between the triggers, feelings or concerns, and the root causes.

Before you can proactively manage resistance, try to determine what resistance might look like. Prosci synthesized responses from hundreds of people to produce the following categories of resistance[16]:

- Emotion: fear, loss, sadness, anger, anxiety, frustration, depression, focus on self
- Disengagement: silence, ignoring communications, indifference, apathy, low morale
- Work impact: reduced productivity/efficiency, noncompliance, absenteeism, mistakes
- Acting out: conflict, arguments, sabotage, overbearing, aggressive or passive-aggressive behavior
- Negativity: rumors/gossip, miscommunication, complaining, focus on problems, celebrating failure
- Avoidance: ignoring the change, reverting to old behaviors, workarounds, abdicating responsibilities
- Building barriers: excuses, counterapproaches, recruiting dissenters, secrecy, break down in trust
- Controlling: asking lots of questions, influencing outcomes, defending current state, using status

Note that, similar to change, resistance is an individual phenomenon. The root causes of one person's resistance are different from another person's because they depend on factors such as personal history, current life events, and other changes that are happening in the work and learning environment. When it comes to resistance to antiracist change there are additional root causes to consider, such as social location, intersecting social identities, privilege, power, and access.

Time expected to complete: 1 hour.

Target audience: Guiding Coalition members.

Purpose of the activity: To design a proactive resistance management plan.

Instructions:

Using Worksheet 6.3, fill out the various sections of the plan:

- Impacted group/project community role. Based on existing evidence, which project community role or stakeholder might be resistant to the antiracist change?
- ADKAR barrier (see Activity 4g: Developing a Communication Plan).
- Resistance anticipated or identified. What type of resistance and when do you think it might emerge?
- How to identify resistance. What will the resistance look or sound like? Name the behaviors.
- Approach for managing resistance. What is the approach? Who will take on what actions?

Activity 4f: Generating Short-term Wins

Even under the best of circumstances individuals will not follow a vision forever, so the Guiding Coalition needs to keep its stakeholders motivated. Short-term wins validate the effort and maintain a level of urgency.[1] Typically they should occur within 3 to 6 months. The project community must see evidence that the change targets are resulting in the desired outcomes, or else they may give up or even join those resisting the change.

In this step, the Guiding Coalition first generates a list of short-term wins based on the tactical plan, tracking system, and strategies. When progress reaches short-term wins, the Guiding Coalition should take time to celebrate. Acknowledging hard work and success is crucial to maintaining momentum for the long-term commitment needed to achieve your vision. Some of the ways you can recognize and reward stakeholders' efforts include[1]:

- offering praise and words of encouragement
- sharing data that demonstrates overall progress
- providing an occasional tangible reward
- encouraging stakeholders to present at meetings and professional conferences
- acknowledging their successes in project communications

- getting institutional leaders to recognize these efforts in broadcast communications, state-of-the-school addresses, and at other major events

Time expected to complete: 1 hour.

Target audience: Guiding Coalition members.

Purpose of the activity: To generate a list of short-term wins or stepping stones to greater opportunities and bigger successes and identify rewards.

Instructions:

- Generate a list of short-term wins. Consider revisiting your tactical plan, tracking system, and integration and acceleration strategies.
- Once the list is complete, brainstorm how to make progress visible and how to reward members of the Guiding Coalition and project community.

Our Experience: Yes!! Small Wins Matter!

Small wins matter. Creating a practice of acknowledging small wins at every Guiding Coalition meeting offered a tangible way to share and learn about progress we were making, as well as provide each other with positive feedback that we were on the right track, even during challenging and highly resistant times. It is important to remember that the wins can manifest in many different ways. Some examples of wins that we celebrated include:

- *when learning an important lesson or finding an opportunity for course correction in the process of trying to achieve a change target*
- *identifying a new ally in the institution*
- *an increase in the number of students participating in the Guiding Coalition*
- *sharing some profound learning from a new book, podcast, or speaker*
- *sharing news of a Guiding Coalition member's new publication or speaking engagement*

Activity 4g: Developing a Communication Plan

Now that your plans are final, it is time to close the loop with the project community. The purpose of this final step is to develop a communication plan that will engage and enable the project community to learn about what is changing (change targets), the phases involved (tactical plan), and how you will track change and be held accountable.

When developing your communication plan revisit the matrix of the Five Levels of Communication as outlined in Chapter 5 (Table 5.2) to ensure that you determine the level (e.g., information sharing, building understanding, identifying implications, gaining commitment, and altering behavior), style (e.g., one-way, two-way, multidirectional, dialogue, introspection), and media or vehicles (e.g., broadcasts, emails, blogs, Q&A, small groups) needed to effectively communicate the change.

We also invite you to consider using the ADKAR model to inform your communication plan. The word "ADKAR" is an acronym for the five outcomes an individual needs to achieve for a change to be successful[17]:

- Awareness – of the need for change
- Desire – to participate and support the change
- Knowledge – on how to change
- Ability – to implement desired skills and behaviors
- Reinforcement – to sustain the change

The model was developed nearly two decades ago by Prosci founder Jeff Hiatt after studying the change patterns of more than 700 organizations. In this activity, consider developing your communication plan to target the *awareness* and *desire* elements of the ADKAR model. For example, for *awareness*, design your initial communications to let people know a change is happening and what type of change to expect. The preferred senders to build awareness are the change sponsor or leaders who can signal that this change is happening and is a priority. For *desire*, share why the change matters and how it benefits to get your people on board with the change. The preferred senders to build desire are managers, mentors, or people who are about to identify the benefits or the "what's in it for me" (WIIFM) for those impacted by the change.

As your change progresses, consider targeting your communications to share information about ways people can gain *knowledge* on how to change; share stories; and share evidence of successful implementation of the desired skills and behaviors *(ability)*. Maintain ongoing communication to remind the project community of the change and what is expected of them *(reinforcement)*.

Time expected to complete: 1 hour.

Target audience: Guiding Coalition members.

Purpose of the activity: To develop a communication plan that informs the project community of your new change targets and plans.

Instructions:
- Use the Engagement and Communication Plan in Worksheet 6.4 to develop a communication plan. Complete this as a Guiding Coalition and/or at the sphere level.
- Implement your communication plan.

Our Experience: Closing the Loop

When our first change targets were determined the Guiding Coalition initiated a broad-based communication plan that leveraged multiple mechanisms focused on building awareness of the change targets and our plan. For example, the Guiding Coalition Change Target Launch Party was an in-person highly interactive experience used to raise awareness about how the change targets were oriented towards addressing racism and bias in medical education. We made use of various types of electronic communications such as emails, newsletters, action updates, and blogs that spoke to the progress and accomplishments of the change targets throughout the course of the year. We added a change target visual tracker on our ChangeNow webpage. We created a digital Year in Review report that is released annually at change target launch events. Products like the report are also important in sustaining our effort because we share them with our Dean (Executive Sponsor), as well as with our Office of Development for future philanthropic cultivation.

REFERENCES

1. Anderson LA, Anderson D. *The Change Leader's Roadmap: How to Navigate Your Organization's Transformation*. Vol. 384. Hoboken, NJ: John Wiley & Sons; 2010.
2. Ahmed S. *The Cultural Politics of Emotion*. Edinburgh: Edinburgh University Press; 2004.
3. David DW, Wilson DC. The prospect of antiracism: racial resentment and resistance to change. *Public Opin Q*. 2022;86(S1):445-472.
4. Okun T. *Characteristics*. White Supremacy Culture; 2020. https://www.whitesupremacyculture.info/characteristics.html.
5. Grosland TJ. An examination of the role of emotions in antiracist pedagogy: implications, scholarship, and practices. *Rev Educ Pedagogy Cult Stud*. 2013;35(4):319-332. doi:10.1080/10714413.2013.819722.
6. Iowa State University. *How to be An Antiracist: Book Discussion Series*. 2022. https://instr.iastate.libguides.com/c.php?g=991417&p=7172640.
7. Reos Partners. *Systems Thinking with The Iceberg Module*. 2015. https://reospartners.com/publications/systems-thinking-with-the-iceberg-module/.
8. Grant-Thomas A, Ogden C, Parker CS. Using systems thinking to address structural racism. Interaction Institute for Social Change; 2014. https://interactioninstitute.org/wp-content/uploads/2014/12/Facing-Race-Handout-actual.pdf.
9. Sevaldson B. *Zip-Analysis: Zoom-Innovation-Potential*. Systems Oriented Design; 2022. https://systemsoriented-design.net/zip-analysis/.

10. Meadows D. *Leverage Points: Places to Intervene in a System*. The Academy for Systems Change; 2012. https://donellameadows.org/archives/leverage-points-places-to-intervene-in-a-system/.

11. Kania J, Kramer M, Senge P. The water of systems change. FSG Reimagining Social Change; 2018. https://philea.issuelab.org/resources/30855/30855.pdf.

12. Levin A. *Climate Cartoon of the Day Domino Cartoon*. CartoonStock. https://www.CartoonStock.com.

13. *Icahn School of Medicine at Mount Sinai*. 2022 RBI year in review report. 2022. https://indd.adobe.com/view/9199547a-61d3-4245-98ae-52e54b548fd4.

14. Grove Tools, Inc. *Graphic Gameplan Leader's Guide - PDF*. 1996. https://grovetools-inc.com/products/graphic-gameplan-pdf?_pos=3&_sid=a21d7aa53&_ss=r.

15. Friedman M. *Trying Hard Is Not Good Enough: How to Produce Measurable Improvements for Customers and Communities*. 10th Anniversary ed KDPamazon; 2015.

16. Prosci. *Managing Resistance to Change Overview*. 2022. https://www.prosci.com/resources/articles/managing-resistance-to-change.

17. Hiatt J. *ADKAR a Model for Change in Business, Government and Our Community*. Loveland CO: Prosci Learning Center Publications; 2006.

7

Phase 5: Implementing and Sustaining Change

CHAPTER OUTLINE

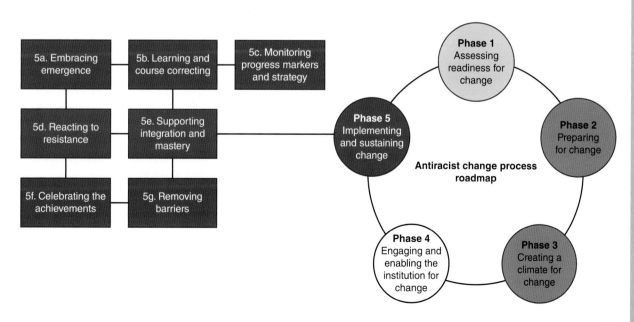

TIME FOR DOWNSTREAM CHANGE

Now that the seeds of a successful change have been sown in the upstream and midstream phases, it is time for downstream change.[1] The goal of phase 5 is to start implementing the change and to embark on a process of integration, learning, and course correcting that will sustain change in the future state. Technically, this phase does not come to an end. Since the change is antiracism transformation, you will be engaging in an ongoing process with no final destination.

Drawing on the work of Anderson and Anderson and others, we will provide detailed instructions on how to participate in seven activities that will allow you to implement and sustain change over time.[1] Where applicable we will share our experiences with the change process. First, we invite those implementing and sustaining the change to consider employing an antiracist practice that is aligned with and can enhance your ability to implement and sustain change over time.

ANTIRACIST PRACTICE: MICROAFFIRMATIONS

Microaffirmations substitute messages about deficit and exclusion with messages of excellence, openness, and opportunity. Powell, Demetriou, and Fisher distilled microaffirmations into a series of tangible actions that can be incorporated into this practice while you implement and sustain change over time.[2]

- *Practice active listening.* Active listening focuses on hearing clearly what is being shared. It can be demonstrated through eye contact, open body posture, summarizing statements, and/or asking qualifying questions to ensure understanding. When implementing and sustaining change, be mindful of active listening behaviors, intentional about creating a culture that employs active listening behaviors, and identify ways to hold each other accountable.
- *Recognize and validate experiences.* Recognizing and validating experiences involves elucidating the what, why, and how. Delve more deeply by identifying and validating the behaviors individuals demonstrate. Respond to their experiences, expressing care about the impact of events and demonstrating a willingness to think through a productive path forward. Implementing and sustaining change requires honest conversations during which participants can share their personal experiences. The facilitators of the activities should recognize and validate experiences. Again, feel free to invite others to employ this practice. This might include:
  - Pausing before speaking. Think about what emotions you are feeling right now: anxiety, insecurity, resistance, anger, shame?
  - Acknowledge and validate. Use words that validate the hurt the other person is experiencing. For example, "You are upset and have a reason to be. I am sorry you had to go through that." "It sounds to me like implicit bias and racism." "This is a hard issue to bring up. I appreciate you trusting me/this group with your anger and sadness."
  - Ask questions to learn more. During the activities, there might be a need to enter into inquiry from a place of care and curiosity, rather than to disprove or contradict. It is important to acknowledge that White people and Black, Indigenous, and People of Color (BIPOC) live different racial realities, thus it might be hard for people to believe something someone else experienced personally. For those who identify as White, notice if your first reaction is to rule out racism or highlight innocent intentions and ask why. If you are a light-skinned person of color,[3] notice if your first reaction is to invalidate or minimize the impact and ask why. Questions could include: "Can I ask you some questions to help me better understand the situation and know how to support you?" "If you are up for it now, could you please tell me more about what happened?"
- *Affirm feelings.* Affirming emotional reactions through verbal acknowledgement can enable the conversation to focus on turning those feelings into actions that will empower, heal, and/or foster learning. For example, "You are not alone." "I can see why that would be hurtful." "I get why you feel that way."

SEVEN ACTIVITIES FOR IMPLEMENTING AND SUSTAINING CHANGE

The activities provided in this chapter are meant to be implemented on an ongoing basis and can be revisited periodically throughout this phase. These seven activities or practices do not need to be completed in order. It is important to consider who needs to participate in the activities associated with each step and the often-absent voices and perspectives that need to be included.

Embracing Emergence

Using the nine core principles of emergent strategy as a guide, the Guiding Coalition and others implementing and sustaining change can develop the capacity to recognize and embrace emergence throughout the process.

Learning and Course Correcting

Learning is vital when implementing and sustaining change over time. The Guiding Coalition can build a formal process for course correction, including a strong case for why it is important, and the cultural norms needed for it to succeed.

Monitoring Progress Markers and Strategy

Monitoring requires tools such as the outcome and strategy journals. These are designed to monitor parallel processes: collecting data about the progress or behavioral change over time (outcome), and the actions or activities when implementing the change toward the future state (strategy).

Responding to Resistance

Developing an approach to managing resistance will allow the Guiding Coalition members to know how they will respond when resistance occurs.

Supporting Integration and Mastery

Being able to recognize what integration and mastery look like will allow the Guiding Coalition and others to support members of the project community and uncover how they can master their part of the new, unknown future state.

Celebrating the Achievements

Waiting to celebrate the new antiracist future is not an option. As incremental change unfolds, the Guiding Coalition must celebrate wins, even if they are small.

Removing Barriers

Implementing change requires the Guiding Coalition and others to anticipate, navigate, and remove barriers throughout the process.

PHASE 5 ACTIVITIES AND INSTRUCTIONS

In this section we outline the seven activities that will help you implement and sustain the change over time, including detailed instructions on how to employ them.

We also provide suggestions for the target audience and the allotted time it might take to complete them. These are suggested guidelines and they should not impede your progress. We recommend that you determine what is needed and how much time it should take to complete the activities based on your institutional priorities. Resist the urge to just "check the box" when completing the activities. We have also provided worksheets that can be used to document and share information about the activities with those involved in preparing for change.

Activity 5a: Embracing Emergence

Now that the initial planning and preparation are complete it is time for implementation, or downstream change. During this phase, the Guiding Coalition will roll out its tactical plans, proactive resistance management plans, and communication plans to achieve the desired outcomes (change targets) of its vision.

For many this will feel like the active phase of the process, when the "real" work happens. As a result, people can get wedded to the plan and try to control how the change is implemented. Be aware that since we work and learn in a complex adaptive system (CAS), there is no formula for how implementation will roll out. Every transformation is unique and subject to the reality of what actually happens or emerges during implementation. Since the environment is unpredictable and chaotic, the Guiding Coalition should not expect the implementation to unfold as planned. It should carry out the plans while continuously learning and course correcting as new information is received. Plans become a starting point of the journey, not the end result. Throughout the process the Guiding Coalition will have to let go of the need to control, focus its energy on being aware of what is happening, and become responsive to events as they arise. The Coalition will rely on strategic and tactical shifts that do not need to be restricted to formal tools or methods for course correction. With this approach, implementation becomes less static or fixed and more of an emergent process. The key is to learn how and when to employ planned (sometimes called "deliberate") versus emergent strategies. In order to do this, the Guiding Coalition must rely on the infrastructure and supports that have been developed in the upstream and midstream phases. Activity 5a will help the Guiding Coalition develop its capacity to recognize and embrace emergence.

Time expected to complete: Throughout implementation.

Target audience: Guiding Coalition members.

Purpose of the activity: To develop the capacity of the Guiding Coalition to recognize and embrace emergence.

Instructions:

- Introduce the nine core principles of emergent strategy and engage in a dialogue by reflecting on the questions provided. Use Worksheet 7.1 to record your answers. We recommend the Guiding Coalition periodically revisit the dialogue and worksheet as needed. It should be noted that embracing emergence might be a new concept that will require a paradigm shift. We advise you to stick with it and see what emerges!

In *Emergent Strategy: Shaping Change, Changing Worlds*, Adrienne Maree Brown offers nine core principles of emergent strategy that can help guide the Guiding Coalition during implementation[4]:

1. *Small is good, small is all – the large is a reflection of the small.* It is often easy for those planning and implementing change to "shoot for the stars," focus on big initiatives, and forget to keep their eye on the small things that truly lead to change. As a Guiding Coalition, how can you keep an eye on what is happening on a small scale, as opposed to just focusing on large scale actions or big wins?

2. *Change is constant – "Be like water."* Change is happening all around you. You are always engaged in a continuous process of change. Thus you must shed a rigid mindset and cultivate an openness to adaptation. To do this, you can draw from the properties of water:

   - Water responds to subtle changes in its environment, such as wind, temperature, and pressure. Be highly attuned to the environment and perceptive of changing conditions.
   - Water is always moving and changing form, even when it appears to be still. Be able to adapt swiftly, and embrace adaptation as a constant.
   - Water flows forward, always seeking out channels of opportunity and following gravity. Be willing to flow with a shared sense of purpose.
   - By shaping the landscape and nourishing life, water is a force of nature. Be agents of change. Be engaged and empowered to collaborate, invent, experiment, and learn. Create a climate of innovation and evolution.

- As a Guiding Coalition, how can you prevent yourselves from being restricted or trapped by your mindset and approach? How can you adapt to certain situations, grow, and change as the transformation unfolds? What are the ways in which you can pay attention to what is happening within the group (with each other) and with the project community? How can you empower yourselves to invent, experiment, create, and learn? What strategies can you imagine that respect the changing nature of change itself?

3. *There is always enough time for the "right" work.* It may not seem possible, but you have the ability to determine what the work actually is and with whom you will do it. Identifying the work has far greater leverage than how one performs it. In all of your interactions there is an opportunity to have conversation that only those people who are present at that very moment can have. Find that opportunity. Be open to deviating from the plan, the task at hand, or the agenda, and embrace what is unfolding in real time if it is aligned with the work of change. As a Guiding Coalition, how can you go where there is energy? How can you be attuned and pay attention to what is trying to emerge?

4. *Never a failure, always a lesson.* Every experience is fuel for creative inspiration. The bigger the failure, the better the fuel. As a Guiding Coalition, how can you turn breakdowns into breakthroughs?[1] What mental models and behaviors must you use to help examine and learn from your failures? How can you create brave spaces to do this?

5. *Trust the people – if you trust the people, they become trustworthy.* Learning how to trust people, and how to allow them to trust you, is a far greater source of leverage than all the productivity tips and tools ever conceived. As a Guiding Coalition, in what ways can you trust each other and those involved in the change? What will this look and feel like?

6. *Move at the speed of trust.* Do not rely solely on the hierarchical structure to propel the change forward. The speed of the Guiding Coalition's change will be determined by how much trust is present, and people will not trust you unless you are vulnerable. As a Guiding Coalition, what are the ways in which you are vulnerable and authentic? What are the ways in which your change target strategies include building trust to accelerate the change?

7. *Focus on critical connections more than critical mass – build resilience by building relationships.* A relationship with the right person can have more leverage than large group consensus. As a Guiding Coalition, what are the ways in which you are actively building relationships with each other and those involved in the change?

8. *Less prep, more presence.* Spending too much time preparing has diminishing returns after a while, while presence brings exponential returns. The sooner you move from preparing to being present, the better the results will be. As a Guiding Coalition, what are the ways in which you can hold yourselves accountable for shifting from preparing to being present? How will you know when you are being present? How can you ensure you are not always on autopilot or relying on the plan to drive your actions?

9. *What you pay attention to, grows.* Another way of saying this is "What you appreciate, appreciates."[5] When addressing racism, many of us have mastered the art of seeing what is wrong, the injustice of the present, and the fault or source of the harm. Critical analysis is an important skill and it also has its limitations. As the transformation emerges, how can your Guiding Coalition balance critique with having an appreciation for what is good and strength based? In what ways can you identify and focus on positive energy throughout the change? Perhaps the actual process of transformational change can help your Guiding Coalition nourish the power of positive vision, hopes, and dreams for an antiracist future.

Activity 5b: Learning and Course Correcting

Anderson and Anderson suggest that successful course correction depends on two key elements: cultural norms, and a mindset that is supportive of learning and adjusting in real time.[1] Drawing from their work, we adapted a process for designing a course correction system that can be used by those implementing the change. This process allows the change strategy team, change process lead, Guiding Coalition, and others to proactively seek information and feedback that tells them whether they are on or off track. The sooner these groups can distinguish the signals from the noise, the sooner they can learn from them and alter course based on their new intelligence, the sooner they will achieve their change targets and unified vision. Activity 5b will help those implementing the change targets build a

formal process for course correction, including a strong case for why it is important and the cultural norms needed to succeed.

The course correction process:
- Hear the wake-up call (recognize a potential indicator that course correction may be needed).
- Discern facts and do not be distracted by the emotions surrounding the potential indicator.
- Check assumptions about the facts.
- Interpret the data.
- Identify insights and possibilities for a new direction.
- Determine the course correction.
- Communicate the new direction.

Time expected to complete: 2 hours.

Target audience: Those involved in implementing the change. This could include the change strategy team, change process lead, Guiding Coalition and other key stakeholders.

Purpose of the activity: To build a formal process for course correction.

Instructions:
- Start by making a case for designing and implementing a formal process for course correction. Those involved in implementing the change should discuss the questions and document answers on Worksheet 7.2 for each category: *incentive*, *risk*, and *burden*.
    - What is our incentive for using a course correction process in our transformation? What are the benefits?
    - What is the risk of not using a course correction process?
    - What is the burden to the Guiding Coalition, sponsor(s), change strategy team, and the project community of using a course correction process?
- Then, establish cultural norms that allow for course correction. Here are some norms for your consideration:
    - Agree to embrace emergence by following the principles as outlined in Activity 5a.
    - Avoid blaming each other for mistakes.
    - Minimize layers of approval in your chain of command.
    - Lower barriers to sharing information across functional areas/spheres/the project community.
    - Increase opportunities to interface and build trust with key stakeholders.

- Allow groups to come together quickly to troubleshoot; do not rely solely on regular meetings.
- Recognize people for positive outcomes and celebrate wins.
- Move forward even if some members are busy or unable to devote time to the change effort.
- To design the system, fill out the Building Your Course Correction System section of the worksheet. Those implementing the change can use the worksheet prompts to brainstorm the plan for gathering intelligence, the process for using that intelligence, and how they will sustain this system.
- The final step is to consider the change sponsor(s) and leaders. Identify how to gain agreement among the sponsor(s) about the importance of learning and course correction in leading the transformational change. Why it is essential to the new antiracist culture of the institution?

Activity 5c: Monitoring Progress Markers and Strategy

It can be challenging to see transformational change in action, especially when it comes to our own behaviors, relationships, activities, or actions. Midway through our change process at Icahn Mount Sinai, we wanted to be more intentional about keeping track of the change that was happening within the Guiding Coalition and with the sponsor. The change process lead wanted to know what was working and not working in terms of the Guiding Coalition's strategy and approach. For example, were the activities and tools effective? Were members aligning themselves to the function and role of the Guiding Coalition? Was the sponsor engaged in their role? Was there overall buy-in to the transformational change process? Were we practicing what we preached? What course correction was needed in our change process? To answer these questions we turned to *outcome mapping*, a structured framework for program design, outcome and performance monitoring, and evaluation.[6]

Outcome mapping focuses on changes in behavior of the people or groups that are influenced by the change. It does not seek to prove causality or attribution for those changes. Instead it attempts to show logical linkages between the changes and the activities, thereby enabling the change to be better understood.[6] Although there are multiple steps to outcome mapping, your outcome and strategy journals are useful tools to monitor

parallel processes: progress markers or behavioral change (outcome) of the Guiding Coalition members and the sponsor, and the actions (strategy) of the change strategy team and the change process lead. Activity 5c can be used by the change process lead and/or change strategy team to develop their own outcome and strategy journals. The journals can also be helpful for members of the Guiding Coalition and other stakeholders in the project community.

Time expected to complete: 2 hours.

Target audience: Change process lead and/or change strategy team.

Purpose of the activity: To develop outcome and strategy journals that monitor parallel processes: behavior change of Guiding Coalition members and sponsor(s), and the actions of the change strategy team and change process lead.

Instructions:

Outcome Journal

An outcome journal is a data and information collection tool for monitoring the progress of the Guiding Coalition towards achieving indicators of behavioral change over time. Worksheet 7.3 is an outcome journal that can be used throughout implementation.

- *Step 1.* Identify an outcome challenge: a statement depicting how the behaviors, relationships, activities, and actions of an individual, group, or institution will change. An outcome challenge is idealistic but realistic. In this case, the outcome challenge is the ideal behavioral change (behaviors, relationships, activities, and actions) of the Guiding Coalition and sponsor(s) that contributes to successfully achieving the change targets and vision. Because changes in people, groups, and institutions cannot be understood in isolation from one another, the outcome challenge can incorporate multiple changes within a single statement rather than breaking them up into separate statements.

Example:
   - Stakeholder: senior leaders/department chairs
   - Behaviors: complete culture shift where equity, diversity, and inclusion (EDI) are prioritized and valued by leaders
   - Relationships: less of a vertical top-down leadership structure and more horizontal collaboration. Better relationships between faculty and staff

- Activities: transparency and accountability; true celebration of diversity
- Actions: decision-making based on cultural values instead of fiscal constraints and incentives
- *Step 2.* Identify progress markers: a set of indicators of changed behaviors of the Guiding Coalition and the sponsor(s) that focus on the depth or quality of the change. Progress markers should advance in degree from:
  - Expect to see = change in behavior that is relatively easy to achieve
  - Like to see = change in behavior that indicates active learning or engagement
  - Love to see = change in behavior that is transformative

  Example:
  - Expect to see = transparency; engagement on EDI topics
  - Like to see = EDI issues prioritized and valued; deliberate investment in EDI activities; hold leaders accountable for their support of EDI
  - Love to see = celebrate diversity; "centering the margins"; EDI becomes core to everyone's mission; change priority away from fiscal implications to culture development
- *Step 3.* Monitor the behavioral change in the outcome journal:
  - Provide a description of the change.
  - Identify the contributing factors and actions.
  - List the source of evidence. This could be observations, data (e.g., survey), one-on-one conversations, meetings, or group discussions.
  - Report on any unanticipated change.
  - Identify lessons and required changes or reactions.

Strategy Journal

Develop a strategy journal: a data and information collection tool for monitoring the change strategy team's and change process lead's actions in support of the overarching antiracist change process. Worksheet 7.4 is a strategy journal that can be used throughout implementation.

- *Step 1.* Indicate the strategies the change process lead and the change strategy team used to execute their roles. This could include strategies related to:

- directing the Guiding Coalition and others towards the desired commitment for transformational change;
- fostering understanding, acceptance, and ownership of the change;
- enabling people to appreciate what they need to do differently to transform;
- adhering to a Results-Based Accountability framework;
- clarifying scope and aligning towards the vision;
- supporting planned change and emergent change;
- engaging in learning and course correction;
- communicating;
- implementing antiracism practices;
- setting the conditions for success;
- managing resistance;
- supporting and giving feedback to the Guiding Coalition and others; and
- modeling desired mindsets, behaviors, and cultural changes.
- *Step 2.* For each identified strategy, document:
- What you did.
- With whom?
- When?
- How it influenced change with the Guiding Coalition and others.
- *Step 3.* Identify the lessons learned and the change or follow up that is needed.

Activity 5d: Reacting to Resistance

The success of implementation primarily relies on the attitude and response of the project community towards the change.[7] Negative attitudes and adverse reactions toward the change may prove harmful—a phenomenon known as resistance to change (RTC).[8] Throughout implementation the Guiding Coalition, change strategy team, change process lead and others implementing the change must engage in reactive resistance management.[9] In other words, they must know how they will react when resistance occurs. It might be tempting to ignore resistance rather than to manage it, especially when it is persistent. While that is tempting in the short term, the end result is predictable. Ignoring resistance can slow down the change process and derail efforts toward transformation.[9] The goal is to uncover the true nature of the resistance. Research suggests that what employees resist is usually not technical change but social change, that is, the change in human relationships that generally accompanies technical change.[10]

Reactive resistance management involves three key components.[9] The first component is to identify the root cause of the resistance. To achieve this, those implementing the change must obtain feedback from those affected by the change (the project community). If anyone is associated with the resistance or has played an active part in the cause, eliciting feedback should be led by an outside facilitator. We recommend offering those affected by the change opportunities to express themselves freely. The purpose of these opportunities is to listen and understand, not to respond.

The second component involves taking action by introducing a range of activities performed by different players, from simply listening and removing barriers, to focusing on the "what" instead of the "how," and offering clear choices and consequences. Examples of actions that can be taken include hosting a series of discussions about the change, and reiterating the case for change (the "why"), what is changing (the content), and how to get there (the process). Give attendees an opportunity to express their point of view and listen to any of their objections. This will help gain mutual understanding by focusing on what can be done to work through these objections, including identifying and removing barriers. It might be helpful for attendees to focus on what is and is not within their control and what they are able to accomplish or create in an effort to move forward. We discuss this in greater detail in the next section.

The third component to reactive resistance management involves enabling and empowering the appropriate resistance managers. While the change strategy team and the change process lead are the conductors of the antiracist change process roadmap, they rarely occupy roles that interact with those affected by the change on a day-to-day basis. During implementation, the most effective resistance managers are the people closest to those affected by the change: managers, supervisors, educators, mentors, peers, etc. It is important to note that resistance management is a role that many people struggle with, which is why it is critical for the change strategy team and change process lead to enable key stakeholders to help manage resistance.[9]

Time expected to complete: Ongoing.

Target audience: Those involved in implementing the change targets.

Purpose of the activity: To develop an approach to reactive resistance management.

Instructions:

Use Worksheet 7.5 to record your approach to reactive resistance management.

- Start by identifying the root causes of the resistance. The goal is to obtain feedback from those affected by the change (e.g., project community). We recommend designing opportunities for individuals and groups to express themselves freely. As a reminder, the purpose of these opportunities is to listen and understand, not to respond. Avoid attempting to communicate resistance away. You will never eliminate resistance by logically and rationally explaining why the change will be good. Unfortunately, people are not motivated to adopt a new antiracist culture just because they see it as "logical." Allow individuals to express their thoughts and feelings about the change. During the feedback opportunities consider questions like these to get started:
  - What is one word to describe how you feel about recent changes?
  - What is working for you or your group right now? What is not? Why do you think that is?
  - What are your hopes? What are your fears? Where do those feelings come from?
  - What do you need in order to be successful?
- After obtaining feedback, revisit the ADKAR (awareness, desire, knowledge, ability, reinforcement) model to help develop corrective actions that can address the gaps.[9,11] These recommendations have been adapted from Prosci[12]:
  - If awareness was the root cause, examine past communications and messages to the individual or group. Create messages that address any gaps in building awareness of why the change is needed. Do you need to reiterate the case for change?
  - If desire was the root cause, assess the incentives or consequences that would create motivation to change. Are these incentives or consequences sufficient? Do adjustments to the incentives or consequences need to be made? Are these incentives and consequences understood?
  - If knowledge was the root cause, examine the opportunities for the project community to

learn more about how to change. Assess the attendance at and effectiveness of these learning opportunities. Is additional education needed? Do current offerings need to be redesigned? Are there gaps in the knowledge and skills being taught?
- If ability was the root cause, personal assistance may be required. What timely assistance is being offered?
- If reinforcement was the root cause, what systems, values, or rewards might help reinforce the change?
- Now, take action by introducing a range of activities performed by different players. In addition to the corrective actions associated with the ADKAR model, those implementing the change can find common ground with those who resist. The goal is to come to an agreement that works for all parties and will help the process move forward. This step may take the longest. Watch for more signs of resistance during this step and try to keep everyone engaged in finding resolutions. Then, take action on whatever agreements were made. Follow through on commitments and intentionally check in to see if the changes that were made are helping. Resistance is rarely resolved quickly. Be prepared to facilitate this process again and make more adjustments as needed (course correct).
- The next step is to activate roles to manage resistance. First, the senior leaders or the executive team help manage resistance by communicating the case for change directly to the project community. On an ongoing basis, are the senior leaders actively and visibly reinforcing the case for change? How can senior leaders help manage the resistance in other ways? Who will help coach the senior leaders on their role?
- Next, resistance managers help manage resistance by working with the people and teams who either report to or work and learn directly with them. Research shows that the best intervention to mitigate resistance comes from employees' immediate supervisors because they know their people best and can work to prepare, equip, and support them based on their unique needs and challenges.[9] When it comes to managing resistance in the project community, it is important to

identify the people who can act as resistance managers. This can be challenging depending on the project community landscape. It might make sense to identify one group that you can prepare, equip, and support in its resistance manager role by focusing on:
- how to have open and honest conversations with those who either report to or work and learn directly with them.
- how to communicate key messages in a way that aligns with the interests of those who either report to or work and learn directly with them.
- how to identify barriers and work to address them.
- how to help people be successful after the change is fully in place.

Activity 5e: Supporting Integration and Mastery

Let us first review the definitions of integration and mastery[1]:
- Integration: "assimilating change so that it becomes the norm. Integration occurs when a person moves from their 'discomfort zone' of *trying* to function in new ways to their 'comfort zone' of being *competent* to perform effectively."[1]
- Mastery: "fully understanding and being competent to fulfill the needs of the new state, continuously developing your skills to new levels of excellence, both individually and collectively. Mastery is a way of being, not a destination."[1]

As an antiracist future unfolds and the project community transforms from the current state to the future state, it is hard to know with certainty what integration and mastery will look like. Below are some examples of indicators of integration and mastery.[1,13,14]

Integration has occurred when you have evidence of:
- Clarifying antiracist work goals, metrics, and expectations for all involved.
- Implementing restructuring to ensure full participation of BIPOC and other marginalized groups, including their worldview, culture, and lifestyle.
- Working to dismantle racism in the wider community, and building clear lines of accountability to racially oppressed communities.
- Operationalizing antiracism across all levels of the institution (e.g., individuals, activities/programs,

courses, units, and community) and with all stake-holders (e.g., administration, trainees, leaders, faculty, staff, students, and community partners).

- Ensuring every individual has adequate skills and knowledge, and the appropriate mindset and attitude, to function effectively and make contributions to the new state.
- Initiating adjustments and course corrections to the new antiracist state.
- Identifying and sharing antiracist best practices and behaviors across the project community, academic medicine, and other health professions.
- Identifying the optimal way of interfacing with others in the project community that promotes inclusion of diverse cultures, lifestyles, and interests.
- Establishing positive working and learning relationships that restore the project community and promote mutual caring and healing.
- Accepting antiracist concepts and terminology and fully exploring the appropriate use of that terminology.
- Internalizing work and learning norms that are antiracist and that combat all forms of social oppression.
- Establishing new norms for power-sharing, influence, and support.
- Clarifying how to communicate with one another, gathering information through different ways of knowing (not just written word), and honoring collaborative and collective knowledge.
- Agreeing on how to manage knowledge and information that honors diverse and interconnected sources of wisdom.
- Agreeing on how decisions are made that reflect full participation and share power with diverse racial, cultural, and economic groups.
- Determining and securing appropriate resource requirements.
- Clarifying how conflicts are handled with inclusive negotiation and resolutions that support peace-building and diversity, especially in the context of deep polarization.
- Creating mechanisms for monitoring and course correcting the mindset, behaviors, and practices of the new antiracist state.
- Leaving behind all nonrelevant practices that cause inequity, fear, violence, harm, and power hoarding. Mastery is occurring when the project community is:
- fully competent in the current state, yet committed to continuous improvement.

- continuously learning and pushing for innovation.
- taking on new challenges.
- mentoring and supporting excellence in others.
- achieving new, more advanced levels of antiracism.

Anderson and Anderson suggest there are two main requirements for people and groups to integrate and master their roles in the new state.[1] First, they must fully understand what it takes to make their role or their part of the institution function effectively on a day-to-day basis. Second, they must understand how their role or their part of the institution fits into and contributes to the larger institution.

Time expected to complete: Ongoing.

Target audience: Those involved in implementing the change targets.

Purpose of the activity: To develop strategies that support integration and mastery across the project community.

Instructions:

Use Worksheet 7.6 to document your strategies that support integration and mastery.

- Review the list of potential integration and mastery strategies:
  - Dialogue and learning groups
  - Workshops, trainings, and follow-up application sessions
  - Coaching and mentoring
  - Identifying and rewarding best practices
  - Working sessions to resolve issues or challenges
  - Conferences to support learning
  - Ensuring the roles and people are linked to the right jobs
  - Appreciative inquiry sessions to fortify what is going well
  - Check-in meetings to bring up operational, cultural, and emotional needs
  - Process or quality improvement work
- Answer these questions:
  - What strategies will you use to support the ability of individuals and teams to uncover how they can master their part of the new state?
  - What are the ways in which you will identify and reinforce integration over time?
  - How will you handle this work with dispersed, hybrid, or virtual teams?
  - How will you ensure that individuals and teams consciously model the new mindsets,

behaviors, culture, and relationships after the launch or "go live" of your change targets?
- How will you make the case to the sponsor(s) to invest in a "whole system" integration and mastery process?
- Revisit as needed.

Activity 5f: Celebrating the Achievements

When we think about celebrating change, we often focus on major long-term goals or milestones. While big wins are important, they occur infrequently and can change over time. We cannot wait for a new antiracist future state to celebrate our achievements. Antiracism is a lifelong practice that is intended to create irreversible change. It is not a destination. As incremental change unfolds we must celebrate the wins, even if they are small. Early in the implementation phase, everyone implementing the change should seek evidence of small wins and achievements that reinforce the change. Consider these ideas when creating celebrations[1,9]:
- Organize ways to publicly recognize groups and individuals. This could include written announcements or special edition newsletters, large group awards gatherings, media coverage, electronic or video celebration address, or town hall.
- Use regular meetings as an avenue for recognition of achievement. This could include putting "recognition" on the agenda (more formal), being spontaneous in the moment, allotting time for peer appreciation, or conducting one-on-one meetings to personalize the message.
- Ensure key sponsors and stakeholders are aware of these achievements. This could include sending quarterly updates to deans and chairs, regularly sharing wins and achievements at institutional leadership meetings, or collaborating with leadership as cosignatories on institutional announcements.

Time expected to complete: Ongoing.
Target audience: Those involved in implementing the change targets.
Purpose of the activity: To develop an approach to celebrating achievements.
Instructions:
Use Worksheet 7.7 to record your answers:
- What methods will you use to celebrate and reward people's efforts to create the new state?
- How can you use your communications and celebrations to further reinforce the mindset, values,

norms, and behaviors required for the success of the new antiracist state?
- How will you ensure that the project community understands the need for further changes?
- How can you reinforce the notion that antiracism is an ongoing process that requires celebration of small wins along the journey?

Activity 5g: Removing Barriers

Throughout the implementation process, anticipating, navigating, and removing barriers is invaluable. Examples of barriers are listed below, but this is by no means exhaustive:
- Leadership: lack of buy-in; change in leadership; a breakdown in relationships with leadership.
- Finances: major challenges in institutional, regional, or federal finances, including major downturns in the nation's economy.
- Attrition and turnover of key members of your transformational change efforts.
- Resistance: active, passive, and passive-aggressive; this can come from any quarter, including people who are key members of your change efforts.
- Shifting political winds: local, regional, national, and global politics that shift attention away from antiracism efforts, including Supreme Court decisions.
- Crises: anything that distracts the institution from sustained antiracism work. Examples of crises include a pandemic, negative press about the institution, natural disasters, and challenges with accreditation.

Time expected to complete: Ongoing.
Target audience: Those involved in implementing the change targets.
Purpose of the activity: To develop an approach to removing barriers.
Instructions:
Use Worksheet 7.8 to record your answers:
- Ask the Guiding Coalition and others who are implementing the change to identify barriers and any potential objections to the change that could be raised. You may find brainstorming and bulletproofing facilitation techniques useful during this first step.
- Select the most serious objections and discuss them using the following questions:
  - Why is this considered a barrier?
  - What impact would it have on the change effort and change targets?

- What could the Guiding Coalition, change strategy team, and sponsor do about it? What would be most effective?
- When should this be done?
- Who should lead which actions or efforts to remove the barriers? Who is responsible or accountable?

It is important to remember that every one of the barriers can lead to a breakdown, and every one of these breakdowns can lead to a breakthrough.

REFERENCES

1. Anderson LA, Anderson D. *The Change Leader's Roadmap: How to Navigate Your Organization's Transformation.* Vol. 384. New York, NY: John Wiley & Sons; 2010.
2. Powell C, Demetriou C, Fisher A. Micro-affirmations in academic advising: small acts, big impact. *Mentor.* 2013;(15). https://journals.psu.edu/mentor/article/view/61286/60919.
3. Hunter M. The persistent problem of colorism: skin tone, status, and inequality. *Sociol Compass.* 2007;1(1):237-254. doi:10.1111/j.1751-9020.2007.00006.x.
4. Brown AM. *Emergent Strategy: Shaping Change, Changing Worlds.* Chico, California: Ak Press; 2017.
5. Gass R. *What is Transformation? And how it Advances Social Change.* 2011. http://stproject.org/wp-content/uploads/2012/03/What_is_Transformation.pdf.
6. Earl S, Carden F, Smutylo T, International Development Research Centre (Canada), Patton MQ, International Development Research Centre (Canada). *Outcome Mapping: Building Learning and Reflection into Development Programs.* Ottawa, ON: International Development Research Centre; 2001.
7. Rehman N, Mahmood A, Ibtasam M, Murtaza SA, Iqbal N, Molnár E. The psychology of resistance to change: the antidotal effect of organizational justice, support and leader-member exchange. *Front Psychol.* 2021;12:678952. doi:10.3389/fpsyg.2021.678952.
8. Folger R, Konovsky MA. Effects of procedural and distributive justice on reactions to pay raise decisions. *Acad Manag J.* 1989;32:115-130. doi:10.5465/256422.
9. Prosci. *The Prosci ADKAR Model.* https://www.prosci.com/methodology/adkar.
10. Lawrence PR. *How to Deal with Resistance to Change.* Harvard Business Review; 2023. https://hbr.org/1969/01/how-to-deal-with-resistance-to-change.
11. Prosci. *The Prosci ADKAR Model - Free ebook.* https://empower.prosci.com/the-prosci-adkar-model-ebook.
12. Creasey T. *How to Diagnose Gaps and Manage Resistance.* Prosci; 2022. https://www.prosci.com/blog/how-to-diagnose-gaps-and-manage-resistance.
13. Philanos. *Resources & News for Philanthopists.* https://philanos.org/philanthropy-resources.
14. Okun T. *White Supremacy Culture Characteristics.* White Supremacy Culture. https://www.whitesupremacyculture.info/characteristics.html.

8

Student Engagement at Icahn School of Medicine at Mount Sinai

CHAPTER OUTLINE

BACKGROUND AND CONTEXT

On the heels of the deaths of Michael Brown in Missouri and Eric Garner in New York in 2014, and the impact of police brutality, racism, and violence on communities of color, medical school campuses remained largely silent and disengaged. Although the Black Lives Matter movement had started a year earlier, the impact of racism and institutionalized violence catalyzed various community organizing efforts across the country. Despite the growing voices from these efforts declaring racism and police brutality as a public health crisis,[1] and the damage to Black communities in particular, the inertia in the medical education community persisted and ultimately sparked dialogue and action among medical students nationally.

Unbeknownst to the leadership of our medical school at the time, a handful of our students coordinated with medical students from two other schools to organize a single, national die-in demonstration protesting racism and police brutality on December 10, 2014, International Human Rights Day. With a commitment to sustain the effort to address racism in health care, the national die-in event catalyzed White Coats for Black Lives (WC4BL) into becoming a formal organization.

Established on Martin Luther King Jr. Day on January 15, 2015, WC4BL was a medical student–run organization that aimed to dismantle racism in medicine and advocate for the health of Black people and other People of Color.[2] The national student movement to address racism in medicine and medical education was born, and included three of our medical students who served as members of the WC4BL Working Group. In their paper published in 2015 entitled, *White Coats for Black Lives: Medical Students Responding to Racism and Police Brutality*, Charles et al. described the organization's priority areas of focus, one of which was a call to action for "medical schools to end their overwhelming curricular and research silence on the history of racism in medicine, address the role of racism in creating disparate health outcomes, and foster strategies for physicians to promote racial justice."[1]

The national die-in protest marked the day our medical school would forever change, and the beginning of our journey to address racism and bias. In an essay entitled *Hand-in-Hand: White Coats for Black Lives* published in May 2015, Dr. Reena Karani (Senior Associate Dean for Curricular Affairs at the time) and Dr. Fareedat Oluyadi (a second-year medical student at the time), each powerfully described the tension between honoring their personal integrity as women of color and complying with the unspoken expectation of faculty not to participate in the protest.[3] Their respective self-inquiries symbolized the journey we would experience as individuals, as a leadership team, and as a medical school with our student body and faculty. Our participation in the national die-in was an inflection point and an explicit reminder that medicine is not immune to the racism that pervades American society.

ANTI-RACISM COALITION: STUDENT-LED MOVEMENT

In 2015, several Icahn School of Medicine at Mount Sinai (ISMMS) medical students formed the Anti-Racism Coalition (ARC) and requested a meeting with the leadership of the medical school, specifically inviting the Dean of the school, the Dean for Medical Education, and the leaders of academic administration, admissions, curricular affairs, student affairs, and diversity affairs. At the meeting the ARC presented the cumulative effects of inequity in the learning environment and a framework for becoming *antiracist*, a term that was new to our lexicon. They expressed their concerns about a lack of diversity, inclusion, and adequate support for students underrepresented in medicine, and the damaging use of race throughout the curriculum. They declared that our educators were ill-equipped to teach about race and highlighted our slow response to contemporary issues related to race, racism, and racial disparities. For each problem area highlighted in the presentation, the ARC also proposed solutions and invited a discussion on next steps for action.

Following that leadership meeting our MD program team initiated a series of discussions with the ARC to review the problem areas they identified and try to navigate their proposed solutions. These meetings were occasionally productive, but more often they were filled with emotions such as disappointment, frustration, anger, resentment, and defensiveness. We never truly overcame the tense and awkward relationship we had with that initial group of students in the ARC. It rarely felt like we were partnering to

address the issues at hand. The students would come prepared to present a litany of problems and complaints. We would listen to each issue, respond with interventions that were already in place or being planned, and commit to addressing the problems with even more effort, energy, and resources, despite never genuinely appreciating how deeply the roots of racism ran.

The stance the ARC most often took was that it was our job to fix these problems, not their job to point out gaps and failings in the learning environment, and certainly not their responsibility to take time away from their studies to resolve the racism. While our leadership team agreed that students were in medical school to be students above all else, there was also a frustration and sense of resentment that students were presenting us with a growing list of insurmountable problems and walking away expecting us to fix them.

To the ARC, the meetings felt like an exercise in futility. To the leadership team these exchanges were exhausting, demoralizing, and overwhelming. The list of problems just kept getting longer, and the nature of the problems could only be solved with more staffing, more money, and more time: in short, more of all the things that we already did not have enough of. In retrospect, we did not have a mental model centered on systems change in order to become antiracist. Instead, our immediate response was focused on the short term. We were grasping for any reason not to face the truth: that systemic racism was deeply embedded in the structures of medicine, medical education, and health care.

One of the first interventions proposed by ARC was to create the space for students to engage in dialogues about the intersection of race, bias, and medicine that would be built into a clerkship rotation and called *Race Space*. Because our diversity affairs colleagues were perceived as part of the problem and were not equipped to lead this specific type of activity, we lacked a skilled racial dialogue facilitator and had to identify an external expert. We identified Leona Hess, PhD: an educator, facilitator, systems thinker, and social worker, whose work was inspired by the notion put forward by Paulo Freire in his book *Pedagogy of the Oppressed* that "Leaders who do not act dialogically, but insist on imposing their decisions, do not organize the people – they manipulate them. They do not liberate, nor are they liberated: they oppress ..."[4] Dr. Hess recommended that our leadership team experience a two-part *Race Space* series. The first part was to experience the session which was being delivered to third year students during the Surgery Clerkship. The second part focused on how we as senior leaders could curb counterproductive activities and behaviors among ourselves so that we could make room for innovation and enhance our capacity to have an ongoing dialogue about racism and bias.

Through this experience and subsequent leadership retreats over the ensuing months, we learned to think of ourselves as fish swimming in the racially oriented/racist cultural waters of academic medicine, completely unaware of the fact that we relied on that water for our thoughts, actions, decisions, and sustenance. We needed to shift our team's mindset towards building the capacity for vulnerability, critical self-reflection, self-awareness of the impact of our actions and words on others, and the importance of centering those who are most marginalized. We needed to reimagine who we were and how we interacted as a team. We also came to see how little appreciation we had for the pain, trauma, and struggles students, staff, and faculty of color endured. Our ingrained habit was to jump to solutions without saying the obvious: I am sorry; this must be terrible for you; it is unacceptable that you should be having this experience.

This breakdown in communication and the breakdown in our relationship with students gradually transformed into a breakthrough as a result of Dr. Hess' coaching.

Our students, particularly those with marginalized identities, needed to feel heard, and as a leadership team we needed to acknowledge the psychosocial impact produced by our learning environment. One aspect of being heard was the importance of documenting in a publicly visible place what students were saying: their challenges, concerns, and pain points. As that list grew and the nature of the issues became more complex and systemic in nature, we realized that this was much bigger than solving isolated problems. Given the deeply embedded nature of racism, our Black and Brown students knew full well that nothing short of a complete cultural transformation would end the racism they confronted every day. We understood that this could never be accomplished in the typical "lifespan" of a medical student: it would need to be our life's work.

Upon accepting this we started our meetings with the ARC by acknowledging how broken our systems were and the role of racism in our environment, and committing to a lifelong process of working on these issues. By definition this meant working at a pace that was going to be slower than expected. We recognized that the manifestations of racism would not be addressed quickly enough to benefit the students involved in ARC at the time, and we apologized for that. We committed to continuing to address pressing or urgent matters in real time; increasing transparency by sharing the list of student concerns with our colleagues and other institutional leaders; creating feedback loops on progress; and engaging in the process of co-creating solutions with students interested in contributing to this work.

Although this approach was not universally embraced by students, over time more and more students came to appreciate that we were being honest, transparent, and accountable for our actions. More importantly, we were able to demonstrate that we believed them and did not question their struggles or approach their suggestions with skepticism. We took it all in and reported back what we could accomplish, provided work plans with timelines for completion, and identified areas where we needed their input or support. For over 2 years, with Dr. Hess now a full-time member of the MD program leadership team, we consistently applied this approach and focused on building a strategy to transform the work and learning environment to be free of racism and bias. This led to the creation and launch of our Racism and Bias Initiative (RBI) in 2018.[6]

STUDENT NATIONAL MEDICAL ASSOCIATION CHAPTER AT ISMMS: ENGAGEMENT AND PARTNERSHIP

A pivotal point in our journey took place in 2020 in the wake of George Floyd's murder. Our Student National Medical Association (SNMA) chapter submitted an open letter to both the hospital and school leadership teams, as did several SNMA medical school chapters across the country, addressing anti-Blackness and racism specific to our institution and in the broader medical community.[7] Akin to the ARC student presentation

5 years before, the call to action remained strikingly similar:

> "Let's be clear: health disparities are a consequence of **racism,** and therefore, that is the issue we have the duty to dismantle. Institutions such as ours can no longer allow either the active or passive propagation of racism in our classrooms, clinics, or laboratories. The Student National Medical Association is not asking for change, we are demanding it. Our **Black Humanity** is, and forever will be, non-negotiable."
>
> **SNMA-ISMMS Chapter Open Letter, 2020[7]**

This time we had a higher level of readiness to receive direct feedback. We were far from our desired aspirational state, but we were poised to use the SNMA letter as a starting point for gaining a better shared understanding of how they prioritized the vast range of issues/requests reported in their letter. We assigned specific tasks to individuals and/or teams, created a triage of timelines, and provided honest feedback to the SNMA leadership team about what could and could not be accomplished.

This point cannot be overstated: we established an open and trusting line of communication with our Black students; we demonstrated in a timely fashion that we were serious about disrupting systemic racism; and all of us, students and administration, were approaching racism with an appreciation that the pace of progress would require a sustained effort, triage, and patience.

We established the first of what would be quarterly meetings that included SNMA student leaders, the Dean, the Dean for Medical Education, and the Dean for Diversity Affairs. The purpose of the meetings was to report on our progress and to get feedback from the students on how we were doing. At our first meeting the students delivered a compelling presentation describing their priorities through a lens of partnership and collaboration, shared understanding, and acknowledgement of the school's previous and current efforts to address racism. The bolded text below from their presentation slides emphasizes the dramatic shift in their tone. This was an acknowledgment that we and our Black students were in this together, were working towards trusting each other, and had a mutual appreciation of how hard it was to be antiracist.

- Shared a clear agenda
  - Introductions
  - Antiracism as a core value
  - **Common objective/goals**
  - SNMA priority areas
  - Discussion and next steps
- Established a shared understanding of antiracism as a core value
  - Creating a safe, equitable environment for *all* students to learn and thrive within
  - Setting the example within medical education by training the next generation of physician leaders to be both clinically excellent and socially engaged
  - Establishing a culture of justice, equity, and well-being
- **Took the time to acknowledge** the administration's hard work and past efforts
- Defined the objectives of the discussion
  - Understand student priorities and **align our shared vision**
  - Establish commitment to data tracking and evidence-based implementation of initiatives discussed
  - Discuss need for resource allocation to carry out initiatives by which **we will collaborate** in future
  - Map out a tentative plan for addressing **mutual priority areas**
- Articulated their priorities
  - Diversity tax: recruitment, hiring, recognition, and promotion (by % Full Time Equivalent or time spent), compensation, active collaboration with affinity groups
  - Diversify patient presentation and address race-based medicine in the curriculum
  - Develop an ethos from the top down that establishes an equity culture

Their final slide posed a question for us that demonstrated just how far we had come in our student–school collaboration:

- What actionable items can **we** expect to see and work on in the next 6 months **together**? 12 months? 3 to 5 years?

The action items from the SNMA letter cut across all of the key functional areas of the medical school including admissions, student support services, curricular affairs, diversity affairs, and medical education administration. The action items were incorporated into the standing agenda of the medical education leadership team (the Strategic Leadership Collaborative) and into the change targets developed by the RBI Guiding Coalition. We subsequently devoted leadership team retreats to further developing and implementing the action plan in partnership with SNMA student leaders who were invited to attend these retreats. Over several months, our collective work resulted in a series of actions that ranged from committing to a regular meeting cadence between the SNMA leadership and the ISMMS Deans leadership teams, to launching robust diverse faculty recruitment and retention initiatives, to establishing formal institutes focused on health equity and antiracism organizational development and strategy, to establishing a number of change targets aligned with action areas from the SNMA Open Letter, such as reviewing the School's mission statement, within the RBI Guiding Coalition.

This partnership with SNMA student leaders had ripple effects far beyond the immediate circle of medical education. Historically we had felt that we were constantly being bombarded with student demands and saw almost no evidence of antiracism as a shared goal. There seemed to be an unbridgeable divide. We often thought that students were being unrealistic, and they often thought we were being disingenuous. This frustration was also felt by the Dean's office, as every discussion with students revolved around things we were not doing well, or were not doing enough of.

The initial meeting with SNMA student leaders was not just an inflection point, it was transformative. The medical education team had seen evidence of this shift, both in ourselves and in students, and we had been working hard to nurture the new dynamic. Suddenly it became clear that we could work on being antiracist as a sustained lifelong endeavor, in partnership with students, and with a shared understanding of how systems, structures, and culture need to change. No more finger pointing, reacting impulsively to crises, or throwing resources at problems without careful reflection and strategic planning.

A PERFECT EXAMPLE

Among the many issues raised in the SNMA letter, one was met with particular skepticism:

> "... compensate student leadership of affinity groups that work directly to dismantle racism including SNMA and LMSA.

> ISMMS should formally acknowledge that soliciting free and/or unpaid advice, education, input and suggestions from Black and AA identifying students in response to white inflicted violence against Black bodies is consistent with white supremacy."

The idea that students should be paid for work that was historically considered an extracurricular activity, done on a voluntary basis and one of the privileges of being in medical school, was unthinkable to many on the medical education leadership team.

In our first review of the SNMA letter we chose not to address student compensation, and yet student leaders had explicitly listed it among their highest priorities. In the past we would have said "no," or said nothing and procrastinated. Instead we tried to listen to the message behind the language. Students were doing a lion's share of the antiracism work at our school, and we were not adequately acknowledging their contributions. So we asked them to tell us more: how might we go about achieving their aims given our initial reservations?

In response, students drafted a well-researched document (*Anti-Racist Medical Student Work*) that laid out a thoughtful, detailed plan with multiple options for recognizing and rewarding their efforts. They shared this document with us for comments and edits, then partnered with us in presenting the concept to the Dean and institutional leadership.

This co-created proposal was approved and launched in academic year 2021–2022 as the RBI × CAP Fellowship,[8] with the primary purpose of expanding the workforce focused on antiracism in our medical school. The Fellowship was so successful that in academic year 2022–2023 we were able to double the number of fellows.[9]

REFERENCES

1. Charles D, Himmelstein K, Keenan W, Barcelo N. White Coats for black lives: medical students responding to racism and police brutality. *J Urban Health*. 2015;92(6): 1007-1010. doi:10.1007/s11524-015-9993-9.

2. *White Coats for Black Lives*. Home Page. https://whitecoats4blacklives.org.

3. Oluyadi F, Karani R. *Hand-in-Hand: White Coats for Black Lives*. in-Training; Published May, 10 2015. https://in-training.org/hand-hand-white-coats-for-black-lives-8775.

4. Freire P. *Pedagogy of the Oppressed*. 30th Anniversary ed. New York and London: Continuum International Publishing Group Inc; 2000.

5. Yeager E. *Common Re-Traumatizing Elements of Institutional Responses to Identity-Based Trauma*. TraumaRoot; Published 2020. https://www.traumaroot.com/resources.

6. Hess L, Palermo AG, Muller D. Addressing and undoing racism and bias in the medical school learning and work environment. *Acad Med*. 2020;95(12S):S44-S50. doi:10.1097/acm.0000000000003706.

7. Addressing Anti-Blackness & Racism at Mount Sinai and the Broader Medical Community: An Open Letter from the Student National Medical Association (Icahn School of Medicine Chapter). *Email communication*. July 1, 2020.

8. Muller D, Willis MS. *Meet the 2021-2022 RBI X Cap Fellows: Change Now*. Department of Medical Education, Icahn School of Medicine at Mount Sinai; Published October 15, 2021. https://changenow.icahn.mssm.edu/meet-the-fellows/.

9. *Meet the RBI X Cap Fellows: Change Now*. Department of Medical Education, Icahn School of Medicine at Mount Sinai; Published October 12, 2022. https://changenow.icahn.mssm.edu/meet-the-fellows-22-23/.

9

Antiracism in Practice: Learning and Development

INTRODUCTION

As discussed in previous chapters, antiracism in practice is the ongoing process of dismantling interlocking systems of oppression and creating new systems of equity with a focus on racial justice. Engaging in this process requires all of us, individually and collectively, to engage in learning and development. As individuals we are influenced by our upbringing and lived experiences, which in turn shape our beliefs, behaviors, and worldviews. It is through personal reflection and continuous learning and unlearning that we are able to change our behaviors and our ways of thinking. This important effort must be supported and reinforced in our work and learning environments. It serves as a foundation for us to understand how racism and bias operate within medical schools and health care systems.

The importance of constantly learning and developing ourselves, especially when we do it as a community, cannot be overstated. We strongly urge your school

to take this on as one of your earliest priorities. It will require humility and trust to admit not knowing, to ask questions, and to invest the time in reading, talking, listening, and watching. It will also demand a great deal of vulnerability to learn from those who have come to our institutions to learn from us: students, residents, and junior faculty, especially those who are Black, Indigenous, and People of Color (BIPOC) and whose voices have historically been pushed to the margins.

At Icahn School of Medicine at Mount Sinai our learning and development have taken several forms, including *Chats for Change, Curriculum Clinic,* and expanding learning to include other institutions, which we will describe in detail in this chapter. These examples are our mechanisms for reaching staff, students, and faculty across the institution, and in the case of National Chats for Change (C4C) and Antiracist Transformation in Medical Education (ART in Med Ed), nationally. Learning and development may take entirely different forms at your school depending on your resources, culture, buy-in and resistance, level of risk aversion, and the degree to which you create a climate that is both brave and safe. We suggest that you let learning and development evolve from your Guiding Coalition, get input from as broad a representative group as possible, constantly collect feedback, and do not be afraid to course correct along the way. Have fun with it, take chances, and above all be responsive to the *people* part of change!

RACISM AND BIAS INITIATIVE: CHATS FOR CHANGE

Importance of Dialogue

The national discomfort with discussing racism and bias racism is a persistent and discouraging roadblock. When we add the widespread "I am not racist" approach that so many people hide behind, it is no surprise that there are few places to formally or even informally talk about racism and medicine. Medical schools have for the most part entered an era where

topics such as social determinants of health and health disparities have become mainstream, albeit not entirely without lingering resistance and efforts to roll back this progress. Now that this beachhead has been established, the next step requires bringing together groups of people to engage in honest dialogue about topics that are more challenging, using words that are harder to say: racism, critical race theory, whiteness, and privilege, to name a few. This is necessary if we are to continue making progress. If we cannot even talk about racism, how are we going to dismantle it and take ownership for creating and contributing to this public health crisis?

In preparing for the kind of dialogue we wanted to have about racism and bias, we devoted a great deal of time to deconstructing and understanding more deeply the types of conversations that typically occur in our work and learning environments. The literature is very clear on the difference between dialogue, which was our goal, and discussion or debate, which is what commonly occurs in committees, teams, working groups, and even one-on-one meetings. Tables 9.1 and 9.2 illustrate some

TABLE 9.1 **The Conversation Continuum**	
DIALOGIC COMMUNICATION VERSUS DISCUSSION AND DEBATE	
Dialogue	**Discussion/Debate**
Seeing the whole among the parts	Breaking issues/problems into parts
Seeing the connection between the parts	Seeing distinction between the parts
Inquiring into assumptions	Justifying/defending assumptions
Learning through inquiry and disclosure	Persuading, telling, selling
Creating shared meaning among many	Gaining agreement on one meaning

From Ellinor L, Gerard G. *Dialogue: Rediscover the Transforming Power of Conversation.* New York: John Wiley & Sons; 1998.

TABLE 9.2 **Why Dialogue?**	
Share insights	Dialogue is necessary in situations where deeper and more widely shared insights into an issue will become paramount for addressing the issue over the long run.
Equalizes power and voice	Dialogue is an investment in bridging differences in ways that do not shut down, or shut out, people with diverse experiences and worldviews. It will not solve all the issues. Still, strategic use of dialogue to help equalize power and voice.
Promotes better decision and sound action	Dialogue is a tool for laying the groundwork for better decisions and sound action because it evolves a diversity of perspectives before attempting to achieve consensus.

From Ellinor L, Gerard G. *Dialogue: Rediscover the Transforming Power of Conversation.* New York: John Wiley & Sons; 1998.

of these stark differences. Typical discussions have a clear, often fixed, conclusion in mind. They tend to avoid uncertainty and vulnerability at all costs. Dialogue, as described by Ellinor and Gerard[1] is particularly well suited to the exchange of ideas and open-ended learning that are required if one is going to create a brave space where people from every level of the institution can come together to address racism and bias.

In Table 9.3, Garran and Miller[2] describe in detail the elements that sustain racism and silence dissent, and the ways in which genuine dialogue serves to strengthen and empower a group of people who have the desire and courage to come together with the hope of breaking through that silence. The items in the left-hand column rely on fear, intimidation, isolation, and an intentional effort to obscure truth and facts. Under Dialogue, the right-hand column offers antidotes to each of these strategies by establishing a bond among people, in our case the students, staff, and faculty who come together to learn from each other.

Chats for Change Design

Beginning in the fall of 2018, the Department of Medical Education at Icahn School of Medicine at Mount Sinai (ISMMS) launched Chats for Change (C4C): a series of dialogues centered on racism and bias in medicine.[4] C4C was based on the notion that dialogue, learning and action are necessary ingredients in order to become antiracist. These sessions were developed in response to demands from medical education staff and students for dedicated time to engage as a community in understanding and addressing racism.

C4C sessions occur weekly and are an hour-long, open invitation to anyone from our school and health system who wants to learn from others' perspectives and contribute their best thinking, in the process revealing each other's assumptions and biases for reevaluation. Attendees explore key concepts and have an opportunity to express themselves based on their own lived experiences.

Each C4C has two facilitators who can be any combination of students, staff, and faculty. A working group of facilitators meets quarterly to determine the themes and specific topics for each season. Examples of themes include:

- Racism 101: A review of key concepts
- Racism in the time of COVID-19
- White supremacy culture characteristics: A deep dive
- In the news: What (happened)? So what (does it all mean)? Now what (do we think, say, do about it)?
- On the Fence: Encouraging divergent views of core concepts

TABLE 9.3 **Why Undertake Racial Dialogues?**	
Racism	**Dialogue**
Racism isolates and silences people, even alienating them from themselves.	Dialogues connect people.
Racism relies on obfuscation and masking privilege.	Dialogue can lead to exploration and revelation.
Racism justifies inequities by alleged genetic or cultural flaws.	Dialogue unmasks these fictions while exposing people to personal stories and experiences.
Racism is a system of power, privilege, and exploitation that benefits one or a number of groups at the expense of others.	Dialogue, even if only temporarily, can establish a level playing field.
Racism marginalizes the voices of people of color while promoting a hegemonic, White discourse.	Dialogue allows all to tell their stories and to hear the narratives of other people.
Racism relies on ignorance.	Dialogue contributes to knowledge.
Without dialogue, racism seems to be the normal state of affairs.	With dialogue, the madness of racism is laid bare.
Racism leads to feeling overwhelmed and resigned to failure.	Dialogue sparks optimism.
Racism divides people and pits them against one another.	Dialogue offers opportunities for cooperation and trust that may lead to collaborative social action.

From Garran AM, Miller JL. *Racism in the United States: Implications for the Helping Professions.* New York, NY: Springer Publishing Company, LLC; 2017.

As outlined in Table 9.4, C4C are always structured in the same way in order to achieve some standardization in the presentations, but more importantly to create conditions that can help establish a brave space for dialogue.

Facilitators use the following sequence at the start of every C4C:

1. Introduce themselves as facilitators and co-discussants, making it clear to everyone that they are not here as experts.
2. Provide a brief history of C4C, including when it was launched and its purpose.
3. Review some grounding assumptions
   - Everyone here is all we need
   - Engage in dialogue, not debate
   - Participate to the fullest of your ability
   - Growth and learning can be uncomfortable
   - Do not be afraid to respectfully challenge one another by asking questions
   - Respect confidentiality
   - Take care of yourself
   - Individuals and organization can, and do, grow and change

TABLE 9.4 Chats for Change Structure

Moving participants through a natural process, from sharing individual experiences, to gaining a deeper understanding of those experiences, to committing to deeper learning and action.

Opening
Welcome participants, explore Who Are We? And introduce dialogue as the agenda and review "What is a dialogue?"

Creating a Container
Creating spaces where there is safety to explore ideas and take risks.

Framing
Framing level sets knowledge and creates a common language for key concepts related to racism and bias.

Dialogue and Debrief
Allowing everyone to be heard and to share their experiences.

Learn and Unlearn Closing
Closing the session by identifying deeper learning and unlearning.

4. Describe the process and agenda of each Chat:
   - Check in: using any interactive audience response system, find out who is in the room (titles and/or roles at the institution)
   - Framing and dialogue: the (non–content expert) facilitators will introduce a topic and offer some framing and context
   - Small group discussion: the audience is randomly broken up into small groups of four to five participants each for more in-depth and intimate discussion
   - Debrief: are there any common themes, insights, or differences to share
   - Learning and unlearning: what did participants learn, or feel the need to unlearn
5. During the framing facilitators strive to interact with the audience as much as possible, in the chat function on Zoom, by unmuting, or by using Slido (our preferred audience response system).
6. Prior to dividing into small groups, the facilitators will remind the audience: (1) that everyone is taught misinformation about people and groups, (2) to not blame ourselves or others for this misinformation, (3) should take responsibility for not repeating misinformation once we have learned that it is not true, and (4) that it is OK to step out of one's assigned small group if the discussion is particularly difficult or triggering (challenge by choice).
7. Breakout group norms are then shared with the participants:
   - Step up, step back: be conscious of taking up too much or too little space, and be emboldened to do something about it
   - "I" statements: speak from your own perspective, not as a representative of any group
   - Name it when it is happening: call our power dynamics when you see them at play
   - Intent does not equal impact: intentions are good, but acknowledge that impact can be harmful nonetheless
   - Challenge by choice: we all have the option of stepping out of, and back into, difficult discussions if the need arises
8. The facilitators offer audience members two to three questions to discuss in small groups. For example:
   - On the fence - Reparations:
     - What would reparations look like in health care? In biomedical research? In medical education? For employees of Mount Sinai?

9. The debrief portion of the session explores common themes and reflections, and asked that small group participants explore the similarities and differences. The goal of the debrief is to ensure that the larger group can benefit from all of the small group discussions.

10. In learning/unlearning, the goal is to encourage continued dialogue and ignite action in the learning and work environment.

In an effort to expand C4C topics and attract a wider audience, we also partner on topics and facilitation with other entities in the school and health system, including student affinity groups, the Office of Gender Equity, the Office of Diversity and Inclusion, Department of Spiritual Care, health system colleagues, and the Adolescent Health Center.

C4C has been a powerful way to engage in critical reflection and dialogue and has attracted over 5000 participants since its launch. It remains the only venue at ISMMS where members of the medical school and health system community can come together to discuss topics that may otherwise be considered taboo. To date, 91% of C4C attendees who responded to the feedback form felt that their session met their expectations, and 92% reported that the facilitators stimulated their interest in the topic. One respondent shared: *"I've felt more comfortable discussing and sharing with strangers my thoughts and experiences with each Chats for Change session."* Seventy percent of respondents thought that the session revealed assumptions and biases that have caused them to reevaluate their thinking. In terms of being able to apply their C4C experience, 85% of respondents suggested that the dialogue will help them make sound action in the future, and 95% said they would recommend C4C to a colleague. Another respondent shared: *"Excellent session today. It was good to have 20 minutes for the breakout rooms. I regularly recommend these sessions to colleagues."*

We made a decision early on not to record these sessions so that participants could feel maximally free to express themselves. As a result, the only way to participate is to be available on the dates and times that C4C occurs. Needless to say, many members of our school and health system community do not have the flexibility to make themselves available, nor does everyone have access to a computer while at work. This is especially true for staff, a cohort that is quite large and more diverse than faculty or students.

Another challenge that we continue to face is attendance, particularly among students. While students were one of the groups that pressed us to create such an opportunity in 2018, very few students attend regularly. There are probably many reasons for this low attendance, including the intense workload of medical school and the time commitments required for extracurricular and career-building activities. While attendance has been a challenge, it is also true that students take ownership of several C4Cs each year, with topics that they select and facilitate. Examples of topics that students have chosen include: Destigmatizing Mental Health Within the AAPI Community; Social Media: A Tool for Racism and Antisemitism; Black and Jewish Solidarity Through the Years; The LANDBACK Movement - Indigenous Rights in Modern Day America; and Mi Cuerpo, Mi Reglas: Reproductive Rights in the Latinx Community.

National Chats for Change (C4C)

In August of 2020, in the wake of George Floyd's murder, we expanded our reach by hosting a national edition of C4C.[5] The format for these Chats is identical to the approach we use internally. Themes have included: Making Good Trouble: Moving From Moment to Movement; Say What You Mean, Mean What You Say; Antiracist Practices in Action; and Cultivating a Community of Practice. Overall, we have received positive feedback about the sessions. For example, an attendee states: *"I would love to expand this program to my school. We have some similar initiatives going on already. I just get so much out of your format."* In 2022, at the request of numerous attendees, we began to offer workshops to train others on the design and structure of C4C to replicate in other medical schools.

THE CENTER FOR ANTIRACISM IN PRACTICE: CURRICULUM CLINIC

Expanding on the efforts of our Racism and Bias Initiative to include the ISMMS Graduate School for Biomedical Sciences, the ISMMS Dean sponsored the creation of the Center for Anti-racism in Practice (CAP) with the goal of integrating antiracism efforts across the MD, PhD, and master's programs and offering additional support and resources in the learning and research environments.[6] CAP was envisioned as a shared resource hub in building the school's capacity to disrupt and dismantle manifestations of racism and bias with

Curriculum clinic journey

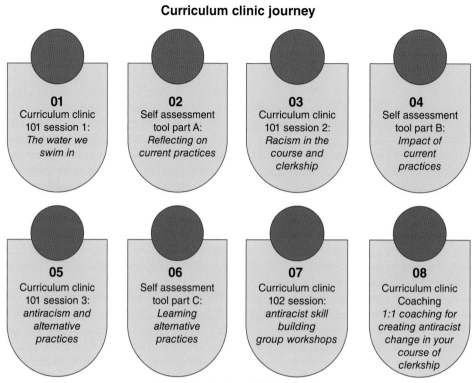

Fig. 9.1 Curriculum Clinic Journey

three areas of focus: (1) antiracist-organizational development and scaling the multiphased change management strategy, (2) equipping faculty educators with teaching and learning design practices grounded in antiracist pedagogy, and (3) aligning current scientific research on race and disease with anti-racist health system-wide initiatives in the learning and research environments. Although CAP has developed innovative programming in all three areas of focus, we would like to highlight *Curriculum Clinic*, a novel program design to enhance antiracist learning and development among course and clerkship directors and teaching faculty.

The purpose of the Curriculum Clinic is to disrupt the perpetuation of racist ideologies and practices in medical education by equipping course and clerkship directors with teaching practices grounded in antiracist pedagogy. The process involves knowledge building, personal reflection, dialogue, and the use of an inquiry-based self-assessment tool and resource guide.

As shown in Fig. 9.1, the curriculum clinic journey is designed to enhance the capacity of faculty to interrogate

the medical education landscape and develop foundational knowledge of antiracist topics, practices, and pedagogy; integrate antiracist pedagogical practices into their learning environments; receive individual coaching; and attend skill-building workshops to tailor this approach to their unique learning environments.

Curriculum Clinic 101: Foundations Series

The first 90-minute interactive workshop, *The Water We Swim In,* explores the history of scientific racism, the biomedical model, and describes how the biomedical model manifests in course/clerkship teaching and learning practices. Participants are asked to identify three ways in which an understanding of the "water we swim in" affects their role as an educator and utilize the assessment tool to reflect on their current practices. After the session attendees are asked to complete the first part of the self-assessment inquiry–based tool to reflect on their teaching practices and self (as educator), self in relation to others (students and faculty), and the larger system within which they work and learn.

The second 90-minute interactive workshop session, *Racism in the Course and Clerkship,* identifies how current teaching and learning practices in medical education perpetuate racism. In this session we identify how racism shows up in the clinical and educational environments and explore the impact of racism in all three domains of the course/clerkship: teacher, learner, and content. The second part of the self-assessment tool is completed after the session by the course/clerkship directors so that they can reflect on the impact of their current practices.

The third 90-minute interactive workshop, *Antiracism and Alternative Practices,* explores antiracism pedagogy and alternative practices that actively address racism and bias in the course/clerkship, as depicted in the self-assessment tool. In this session we describe the concepts of antiracism, antiracist pedagogy, and antiracist practices related to the teacher, learner, and content. A resources guide accompanies this session and includes actionable steps to help integrate antiracism practices that focus on behaviors the teacher or educator can demonstrate, the learning environment that can be cocreated, and the content that can be delivered.

Examples of antiracist pedagogy include:

Focusing more on collaboration and community than individualism, competitiveness, and authority

Enhancing one's awareness of how history, politics, and social identity impact learning, working, power relations, and the generation of new knowledge

Exploring how race as a socio-political construct impacts everyone who is a member of a group that experiences bias

Seeing oneself as an integral part of what is being taught, learned, and practiced

As of March 2023, 86% of course and clerkship directors have participated in the series. Feedback has been overwhelmingly positive, with over 90% of respondents agreeing or strongly agreeing that the clinics provided the tools, skills, and/or knowledge necessary for their course/clerkship. Over 90% agreed that the design of the sessions encouraged participation and interaction, reinforced a deep understanding of the material, and that the pace of the sessions allowed them to comprehend and process the information. As of this writing we are in the process of providing one-on-one coaching sessions to reinforce the session content and to help course and clerkship directors implement antiracist practices, as outlined in the guide.

Curriculum Clinic 102: Skill Building Series

In this series, faculty educators are equipped with antiracist pedagogical practices to integrate into their respective learning environments. Participation in this series is not mandatory. As shown in Table 9.5, workshop topics include setting group norms, antiracist bedside teaching, and managing racist behaviors from patients, all of which provide faculty with the practical skills to operationalize alternative practices in their respective learning environments. We completed our first cycle of the Curriculum

TABLE 9.5 Curriculum Clinics 102: Workshop Topics and Learning Objectives	
Session Title	**Learning Objectives**
Setting norms for inclusive learning environments Setting norms for inclusive clinical learning environments	• Describe ways in which my lived experiences and identities contribute to the culture of my clinical learning environment. • Identify concrete strategies and techniques that foster liberating clinical learning environments. • Apply these strategies and techniques within my role as clerkship director or clerkship faculty.
Antiracist clinical teaching skills at the bedside	• Identify examples of racist norms in the clinical environment. • Describe techniques to counter these norms to improve patient care and student education. • Apply these strategies and techniques within your role as a clinician educator.
Responding to racist behaviors from patients	• Identify examples of racist and other discriminatory behavior from patients/caregivers in the clinical environment. • Describe examples of racist and other discriminatory behavior from patients/caregivers in the clinical environment. • Apply these strategies and techniques within your role as a clinician educator.

Clinic 102 series in February 2023. Twenty course and clerkship directors and faculty participated. 100% of attendees reported that they received the specific skills they needed to implement changes and were planning to do so.

ANTIRACIST TRANSFORMATION IN MEDICAL EDUCATION

As we describe at length in this book, dismantling racism in medical school settings requires a strategy that is broadly transformative, ongoing, people dependent, and responsive to the world around us.

After establishing our approach to antiracism, and with several years of experience under our belt, we submitted a proposal for a grant that would fund the dissemination of this approach to medical schools in the United States and Canada. We saw this as an opportunity to extend learning and development beyond our four walls by building the capacity of other schools to harness the power of transformational change; establishing a community of practice whose members could learn and develop together; and allowing us to learn from the richness of experiences among our peers.

In October of 2021, the Josiah Macy Jr. Foundation funded ART in Med Ed, a 3-year project to disseminate ISMMS's change-management strategy at 11 partner medical schools in North America.[7]

The aims of the project include:

1. *Capacity development.* Developing the capacity of medical schools to dismantle systemic racism and bias in their work and learning environments by implementing a multiphased change management strategy.
2. *Community of practice.* Promoting shared learning on how to dismantle racism within and across medical schools using systems change tools and processes.
3. *Replicable and scalable.* Determine the conditions in which ISMMS's transformational change strategy could be replicated at other medical schools, and identify which of its features yield the best outcomes in order to disseminate it to a larger number of medical schools.

Six Core Competencies

ART in Med Ed was designed to focus on six core competencies that build upon a school's existing capacity (skills, knowledge, and behaviors). The goal of these competencies was to promote transformational change at, and establish a community of practice (Table 9.6) among, the participating schools.

Application Process

Co-creation was a central tenet of ART in Med Ed, and necessary to deconstruct power dynamics, foster meaningful relationships, and involve multiple stakeholders who would actively contribute to the process of change. In our request for applications we selected schools that expressed interest in addressing racism and bias; demonstrated an openness to learning and implementing a transformational-change strategy; and were committed to fielding a diverse cohort of leaders, faculty, students, and staff to actively participate in a multiyear collaboration.

TABLE 9.6 ART in Med Ed's Core Competencies	
Competency 1 | Challenge the Current State	• Gather and analyze feedback and data. • Help build a business case for why change is imperative. • Establish a sense of urgency. • Determine organizational readiness for change.
Competency 2 | Harmonize and Align Stakeholders	• Build trust and confidence in people at all levels of the work and learning environment. • Differentiate change management roles. • Select members for, and build, a Guiding Coalition. • Coach leaders about their sponsorship role. Facilitate a process that will create a compelling change vision. • Help design a change management communication plan using the ADKAR model.
Competency 3 | Activate Commitment	• Obtain buy-in to the vision. • Define and anticipate reactions to change. • Build critical mass.
Competency 4 | Nurture and Formalize a Strategy	• Identify and implement change targets that address systems issues. • Use a results-based accountability approach to select appropriate metrics. • Use a variety of implementation and planning tools.

TABLE 9.6 ART in Med Ed's Core Competencies—cont'd	
Competency 5 | Guide Implementation	• Foster collaboration between diverse groups. • Utilize organizational politics positively. • Identify motivational factors for a broad spectrum of individuals. • Use short-term wins to build momentum. • Develop change targets/efforts towards systems change.
Competency 6 | Evaluate and Institutionalize the Change	• Create a process to evaluate the change targets. • Identify ways to institutionalize the change. • Create a change-ready organization. • Implement a process for course correction. • Monitor outcomes (behaviors) and strategy.

ADKAR, Awareness, desire, knowledge, ability, and reinforcement; *ART in Med Ed,* Antiracist Transformation in Medical Education.

Candidate schools were asked to address the following questions in their application:

1. Address why your institution is uniquely positioned to participate in our collaboration and learning platform.
2. Provide a list of existing programs, offices, staff, and resources that address racism and bias at your institution.
3. Define the process for ensuring the cohort of participants will include a diverse group, including faculty, staff, leaders, and students.
4. Provide a letter of support from the Dean demonstrating the institution's long-term commitment to carry out this work.
5. Provide a letter of support from student leadership demonstrating their long-term commitment to carry out this work.

Selection Process

We received applications from 48 schools (Table 9.7). The selection committee was composed of 22 staff, students, and faculty who represented a broad spectrum of our medical school stakeholders and had demonstrated sustained, active participation in antiracist efforts. A complete list of the committee member roles and titles can be found in Appendix 9.1.

Each application was reviewed by three committee members who ranked the applications based on a standard rubric developed for this purpose. Once each application was ranked, selection committee members met to discuss and reconcile their scores. Once the scores were determined, instead of selecting the top-ranked schools we intentionally selected schools across the full spectrum of rubric scores, paying close attention to include the most diverse geographic locations, types of school, years founded, and current activities and

TABLE 9.7 ART in Med Ed Applicant and Selected Schools Demographics		
Demographics	**Applied**	**Selected**
Total Number, N	48	11
School Type, N (%)		
Public	32 (66.7)	7 (63.6)
Private	15 (31.2)	4 (36.4)
Federal	1 (2.1)	0 (0.0)
Program Type, N (%)		
MD	46 (95.8)	10 (90.9)
DO	2 (4.2)	1 (9.1)
Established, N (%)		
1700s	1 (2.1)	1 (9.1)
1800s	16 (33.3)	3 (27.3)
1900s	22 (45.8)	5 (45.4)
2000s	9 (18.6)	2 (18.2)
Enrollment Size, N (%)		
<100	1 (2.1)	0 (0.0)
101–500	21 (43.7)	6 (54.5)
501–1000	21 (43.7)	4 (36.4)
>1000	5 (10.4)	1 (9.1)
Application Scores, Mean (SD)	8.25 (1.00)	8.96 (0.53)

ART in Med Ed, Antiracist Transformation in Medical Education; *SD,* standard deviations.

resources dedicated to addressing racism. The goal of this approach was to give us a deeper understanding of institutional conditions that would yield the best possible change management outcomes and be replicable at other medical schools.

APPENDIX 9.2   Committee Member Roles

Associate Dean, Undergraduate Medical Education
  Affairs
Change Management Strategy Project Manager
Communications and Marketing Manager
Dean for Medical Education
Director of Student Financial Services
Education Program Manager
Education Program Manager-MSH
Executive Assistant, Dean for Medical Education
Faculty
Integration Program Manager
Process Improvement and Strategy Program Manager
Senior Associate Dean for Diversity and Inclusion in
  Biomedical Education
Senior Associate Dean for Medical Education
  Administration
Senior Coordinator
Senior Director of Strategy and Equity Education
  Programs
Senior Global Health Program Coordinator
Six students

We selected the following 11 medical schools:
- Brody School of Medicine, East Carolina University
- College of Medicine, University of Saskatchewan
- Columbia University Vagelos College of Physicians and Surgeons
- David Geffen School of Medicine at the University of California, Los Angeles
- Duke University School of Medicine
- The George Washington University School of Medicine and Health Sciences
- The Ohio State University College of Medicine
- University of Arizona College of Medicine - Phoenix
- University of Minnesota Medical School
- University of Missouri-Columbia School of Medicine
- University of the Incarnate Word School of Osteopathic Medicine

Expectations

Each of the 11 selected schools identified up to 15 cohort members and one to two project leads who would serve as the main point of contact for their cohort. Project leads were responsible for maintaining communication, coordinating program activities, and supporting the implementation of ART in Med Ed in their institution. Among all schools, cohort members included faculty, staff, and students across multiple functional areas and departments.

All cohort members were expected to actively participate in:
- Guiding stakeholder groups and individuals towards the desired commitment for change necessary to transform medical education.
- Fostering understanding, acceptance, and ownership of the change within their institution.
- Enabling people to appreciate what they need to do differently to transform from the current state to the unknown future state.
- Developing and implementing a multiphased change management strategy and ensuring content, people and process elements of the change are all aligned.
- Monitoring behavioral change (outcome mapping) and strategy implementation.
- Course correcting along the way to constantly align their strategy towards antiracism transformation.

Capacity Building Model

We adapted the Change Process Roadmap based on the work of Anderson and Anderson,[8] and Kotter,[9] as outlined, with modifications, in Chapters 3 to 7 of this book. The ART in Med Ed cohorts progressed through the five phases of transformational change, each of which had self-directed learning activities. Within each phase, the capacity development design involved five stages: framing and dialogue session, self-directed learning activities, coaching session, community of practice session, and evaluation (Table 9.8).

TABLE 9.8 **Capacity Development Stages**	
Framing and Dialogue	Work with each cohort to build group cohesion and provide instruction on critical content. This serves as a foundation for the tools and processes that will be introduced during the self-directed learning stage. These 1.5-hour sessions are live online via Zoom.
Self-directed Learning	Cohort members engage in self-directed learning that level-sets knowledge and introduces new change management strategy tools and processes.
Coaching	Provide *Systems Change* coaching to each school's cohort, with separate coaching sessions for students to map outcomes and/or monitor the strategy over time. These 1.5-hour sessions are live online via Zoom.
Community of Practice	All cohorts come together to share practices and create new knowledge to dismantle racism and transform medical education. These 1.5-hour sessions are live online via Zoom.
Evaluation	Participants are prompted to take a brief survey that provides feedback on the content, facilitation methods, and learning platform.

REFERENCES

1. Ellinor L, Gerard G. *Dialogue: Rediscover the Transforming Power of Conversation.* New York: John Wiley & Sons; 1998.
2. Garran AM, Miller JL. *Racism in the United States: Implications for the Helping Professions.* New York, NY: Springer Publishing Company, LLC; 2017.
3. Okun T. *Characteristics.* White Supremacy Culture. https://www.whitesupremacyculture.info/characteristics.html.
4. Icahn School of Medicine at Mount Sinai. *Chats for Change: Mount Sinai.* 2023. https://changenow.icahn.mssm.edu/chatsforchange/.
5. Icahn School of Medicine at Mount Sinai. *Change Now: Creating a Climate for Change.* 2023. https://changenow.icahn.mssm.edu/national-chats-for-change/.
6. Icahn School of Medicine at Mount Sinai. *Center for Antiracism in Practice.* https://icahn.mssm.edu/about/diversity/center-for-antiracism.
7. Icahn School of Medicine at Mount Sinai. *Antiracist Transformation in Medical Education.* https://icahn.mssm.edu/education/medical/antiracist-transformation.
8. Anderson LA, Anderson D. *The Change Leader's Roadmap: How to Navigate Your Organization's Transformation.* Vol. 384. New York, NY: John Wiley & Sons; 2010.
9. Kotter JP. *Accelerate!* Harvard Business Review; 2012. https://hbr.org/2012/11/accelerate.

Antiracist Community of Practice

INTRODUCTION

Let us dream into the future for a moment. Imagine that we have transformed our culture from being systemically racist and inequitable to antiracist and just. We have successfully created conditions for an inclusive, thriving community. We have applied new knowledge and adopted innovative approaches that have transformed the way we work and learn together. We have shifted paradigms to embrace power sharing, co-creation, participatory decision-making, and equitable outcomes. Although this is a dream, it provides a vision for what we can build together, lifting us out of the intractable problems of racism and bias. If we are going to align ourselves with this aspirational future state, it will require a community of people who come together to learn, share, and build our collective capacity to achieve this dream.

In this chapter, we review the concept of community of practice (CoP) and describe it in the context of antiracist medical education. We also discuss our experience in developing a CoP with 11 medical schools in North America as part of our grant-funded Anti-Racist Transformation in Medical Education (ART in Med Ed) program.

COMMUNITY OF PRACTICE

There are many ways people come together to learn and develop knowledge as a group, community, or organization. Collective learning has occurred throughout history, whether rooted in cultural traditions and practices of information sharing and relationship building (e.g., oral histories and online communities), or the formal and informal learning pathways in community, work, and academic settings (e.g., professional and faculty development, academic associations, professional organizations, and networking).

Cognitive anthropologists Lave and Wenger first characterized the phenomenon of collective learning as a CoP: a group of people who share a concern or a passion for something they do and learn how to do it better as they interact regularly.[1] As shown in Fig. 10.1, this definition reflects three key characteristics of a CoP: domain, community, and practice.[2]

1. *Domain.* Community members have a shared domain of interest, competence, and commitment that distinguishes them from others. This shared domain creates common ground, inspires members to participate, guides their learning, and gives meaning to their actions.

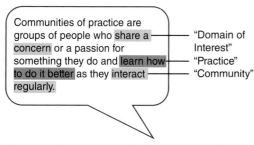

Communities of practice are groups of people who share a concern or a passion for something they do and learn how to do it better as they interact regularly.

— "Domain of Interest"
— "Practice"
— "Community"

Fig. 10.1 Characteristics of a Community of Practice

2. *Community.* Members pursue this interest through joint activities, discussions, problem-solving opportunities, information sharing, and relationship building. The notion of a community creates the social fabric for enabling collective learning. A strong community fosters interaction and encourages a willingness to share ideas.

3. *Practice.* Community members are actual practitioners in this domain of interest and build a shared repertoire of resources and ideas that they take back to their practice. While the domain provides the general area of interest for the community, the practice is the specific focus around which the community develops, shares, and maintains its core of collective knowledge.

As outlined in Table 10.1, a CoP can serve many functions. Based on these functions, it is evident that CoPs are people dependent. The true value of this approach is in the depth of the participants' reflection and inquiry, and how they put co-created knowledge into action.[3]

A community takes time and dedication to grow and evolves through various stages during its lifetime. Table 10.2 illustrates the progression of the stages.

In the *potential state*, the CoP is a loose network of people who have common interests around a key issue.

TABLE 10.1	**Functions of a Community of Practice**
Filtering	Organizing and managing information that is worth paying attention to.
Amplifying	Taking new, little-known, or little-understood ideas, giving them weight and clarity, and making them more widely appreciated.
Investing and providing	Giving each other the resources and support needed to implement the change-management strategy.
Convening	Bringing together participants to promote collaboration between and across institutions.
Community building	Promoting and sustaining collective values and standards.
Learning and facilitating	Helping each other implement strategies, tools, and processes more efficiently and effectively.

From Wenger-Trayner E, Wenger-Trayner B. *Introduction to Communities of Practice.* 2015. https://www.wenger-trayner.com/introduction-to-communities-of-practice/.

TABLE 10.2	**Five Stages of Community of Practice**
Potential	A loose network of people recognizes common interests around a key issue.
Coalescing	The community establishes the value of sharing knowledge and develops relationships and sufficient trust.
Maturing	The community clarifies its focus, role, and boundaries. Shifts from sharing tips to developing a body of knowledge.
Stewardship	The community must maintain its relevance and its voice, keep the tone and focus lively and engaging, and keep itself on the cutting edge.
Transformation	Communities naturally transform or die. Sometimes communities split into new communities, or they merge with other communities. Sometimes they lose relevance and die.

From Wenger E. *Communities of Practice: Learning as a Social System. The Systems Thinker.* 2017. https://thesystemsthinker.com/communities-of-practice-learning-as-a-social-system/.

The pitfall of this stage of a CoP is that it is common and can exist in a variety of settings, but may never evolve beyond this stage if the members involved do not establish a value for knowledge sharing.

A CoP at the *coalescing* stage establishes the value of sharing knowledge and develops relationships and sufficient trust. This stage is a tipping point towards becoming a *maturing* CoP. During the *coalescing* stage the CoP interrogates its current and future states by deciding how it wants to function and reflecting on what it may need to coalesce as a group.

The pivot from the coalescing stage to the maturing stage signifies a growing sense of ownership over a body of knowledge and expertise. The last two stages of *stewardship and transformation* speak to the creation of conditions that allow for a thriving CoP, enabling it to develop the strategies to stay relevant and apply knowledge while also leaving open the possibility of transforming into a new community or accepting its completion as a CoP. A CoP that pivots towards *stewardship* can support steady, relevant, and long-lasting systems change, shifting the conditions that are holding the problem in place.[4]

A CoP can be leveraged because it provides both short- and long-term value for individual members and organizations as shown in Table 10.3. For example, the short-term value for individual members may be realized in the *potential* stage for those who are new and willing to participate in the transformational change process to mitigate against isolation. For organizations the CoP can serve in the short term as a partner in thinking and planning. Long term, the value for individual members may manifest as a sustained, robust personal and professional capacity to participate in and lead transformational change. For organizations a CoP can create the space for ongoing innovation and for becoming a seasoned *steward* of knowledge, practice, and strategy.

Finally, a CoP is entirely people dependent. The true value of this approach to collective learning is in the depth of the participants' reflection and inquiry, and how they put co-created knowledge into action.[3] The Ask, Learn, and Share model, shown in Fig. 10.2, may accelerate the coalescence of the CoP by determining how an individual, group, and community behave to deepen the value of shared knowledge and trusted relationships.

The first reference linking the concept of CoP to medicine and medical education appeared in 2002.[4] It has since been referenced as a theoretical learning model used in undergraduate medical education, postgraduate education, and continuing professional development.[4] The concept of CoP has also been used as an effective model for achieving quality outcomes in health care.[4-6] Given the history and successful implementation of CoPs in the field, it seems fitting to create an antiracist CoP where a group of individuals or institutions come together to actively learn, share knowledge, and engage in collaborative efforts to dismantle racism and promote equity and justice.

TABLE 10.3 **Why Focus on Communities of Practice?**		
	For Members	**For Organizations**
Short-term value	• help with challenges • access to expertise • confidence • fun with colleagues • meaningful work	• problem solving • time saving • knowledge sharing • synergies across sectors/districts • reuse of resources
Long-term value	• personal development • enhanced reputation • professional identity • networking	• strategic capabilities • keeping up-to-date • innovation • retention of talent • new strategies

From Edmonton Regional Learning Consortium. *Why Communities of Practice are Important. Community of Practice.* 2016. https://www.communityofpractice.ca/background/why-communities-of-practice-are-important/.

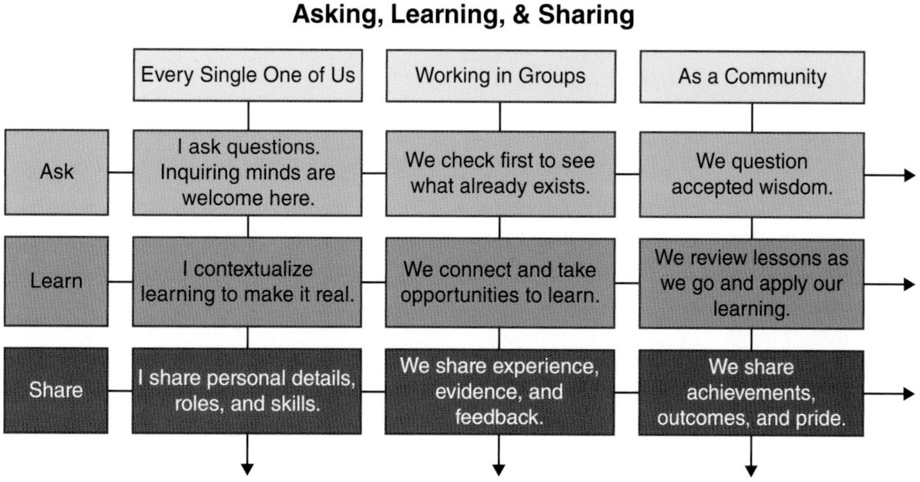

Asking, Learning, & Sharing

Fig. 10.2 Ask, Learn, Share Model

ART IN MED ED CoP

One of the three aims of ART in Med Ed is to promote shared learning on how to dismantle racism within and across medical schools using systems change tools and processes.[6] To meet this aim, we invited the 11 participating medical schools to participate in a CoP, creating sustained accountability and connections, expanding beyond siloed departments and institutions, and developing new ways of collaborating and cross-pollinating ideas and practices.

When we first started ART in Med Ed we held CoP sessions at the end of each program phase so that all the school cohorts could learn new knowledge and skills from each other, and implement them in their respective work and learning environments. As we entered phase 3 of the program in May 2022, in response to the desire of the participating schools we course-corrected and began to host monthly CoP virtual sessions with all the participating medical schools. There was a desire to meet more frequently and the topics were generated by the participants, not the program administrators.

The CoP sessions have evolved over time. Each CoP session includes self-selected breakout sessions based on relevant topics. These have included:

- *Developing the Guiding Coalition.* What is working well for your Guiding Coalition? Are there aspects to improve upon? Are there any barriers that you anticipate moving forward? How are you recruiting Guiding Coalition members? What tools, resources, and communications have been implemented or are intended to be implemented?
- *Adopting transformational change management tools.* Are there existing projects/efforts that could benefit from using the transformational change management tools? What are some of the actions you or others might take to encourage more people to support the implementation of the tools at your institution?
- *Centering student involvement.* How have students been incorporated into your antiracist practices? How could student involvement be better supported?
- *Supporting group structure.* How have you dealt with changes to the structure and attendance of your project community members?
- *Individual and group support.* Any tips on how to support yourself and the project community when people are feeling overwhelmed and burned out?
- *Developing advocacy.* What are some ways to advocate for more support for antiracist work, such as protected time?
- *Developing your project community.* How have you decided who is "in" and who is "out" of your project community?
- *Encountering barriers.* Are there barriers, setbacks, and challenges getting in the way of the work?
- *Developing communications.* How have you approached getting buy-in from stakeholders and potential Guiding Coalition members? What has worked? What could be improved?

- *Implications of D/E/I legislation.* Have you or your institution encountered barriers related to anti-Diversity, Equity, and Inclusion (D/E/I) legislation? How has your institution dealt with this? What could be done as a CoP that you cannot accomplish as a single institution?

The ART in Med Ed CoP continues to mature. Its members continuously clarify the focus of the CoP based on where the schools are in the process of implementing transformational change and what is happening in their work and learning environments. The CoP also provides opportunities for leaders among these schools to have a hand in convening the group and generating the areas of focus. These developments are important reminders that there is no known destination or fixed endpoint in becoming antiracist. Instead, the focus is on continuous progress, making the most of emerging opportunities, and transforming breakdowns into breakthroughs along the way.

We invite you to join us on this journey and look forward to supporting you along the way.

REFERENCES

1. Wenger-Trayner E, Wenger-Trayner B. *Introduction to Communities of Practice.* Wenger-Trayner; Published June 2015. https://www.wenger-trayner.com/introduction-to-communities-of-practice/

2. Edmonton Regional Learning Consortium. Creating Communities of Practice. *What is a Community of Practice?* Community of Practice. https://www.communityofpractice.ca/background/what-is-a-community-of-practice/#:,:text=Cognitive%20anthropologists%20Jean%20Lave%20and,acts%20as%20a%20living%20curriculum.

3. Edmonton Regional Learning Consortium. *Why Communities of Practice are Important.* Community of Practice; 2016. https://www.communityofpractice.ca/background/why-communities-of-practice-are-important/.

4. Kania J, Kramer M, Senge P. *The Water of Systems Change.* FSG – Reimagining Social Change; 2018. https://philea.issuelab.org/resources/30855/30855.pdf.

5. Wenger E. *Communities of Practice: Learning as a Social System.* The Systems Thinker; 2017. https://thesystems-thinker.com/communities-of-practice-learning-as-a-social-system/.

6. Icahn School of Medicine at Mount Sinai. *Anti-Racist Transformation in Medical Education.* https://icahn.mssm.edu/education/medical/anti-racist-transformation.

Appendix

WORKSHEET 3.1   Activity 1b: Sponsor Readiness Assessment: Sponsor Readiness
Are your sponsors:
Aware of their importance in making change successful?
Aware of their biggest roles in supporting the project?
Active and visible throughout the change initiative?
Building the coalition necessary for change to be successful?
Communicating directly and effectively with people who will be impacted?
Aware that the biggest mistake is failing to personally engage as the sponsor?

Continued

WORKSHEET 3.1   Activity 1b: Sponsor Readiness Assessment: Sponsor Readiness—cont'd

Prepared to manage resistance?

Prepared to celebrate successes?

Setting and reconciling clear priorities regarding this change, other initiatives and day-to-day work?

Avoiding the 'flavor of the month' syndrome?

As a group, reflect on the following:

What are your initial thoughts/reactions to the answers?

What are the answers that surprised you and should be reexamined? Why? Is there something not being said?

What are the next steps in getting the sponsors ready and selecting them (if not already selected)

How will sponsors engage throughout the life of the change process?

Adapted from Prosci. *Primary Sponsor's Role and Importance*. Prosci. https://www.prosci.com/resources/articles/primary-sponsors-role-and-importance.

WORKSHEET 4.1   Activity 2a: Identifying Your Project Community

Project Community Questions

1. Which stakeholders (internally and externally) should be included in this antiracist transformational change effort?

2. Is everybody who must have a voice in this transformation identified and ready to have input as the change is being planned?

3. How will this change effort interface with other projects underway?

4. What are the best ways to inform stakeholders that they are an important part of this effort's project community? Think about the type of message and communication method (e.g., meetings, events, emails, etc.).

5. What will you ask the various members of the project community to do now to motivate them to act? What is the "call to action?"

6. How will you use the project community to inform all the phases of the change process roadmap?

Continued

WORKSHEET 4.1   Activity 2a: Identifying Your Project Community—cont'd

Members of Your Project Community	Identify the members of your project community for your change effort. Name the key players from the following groups:
Stakeholder groups or individuals	
Functional areas of school/institution	
Locations within school/institution	
Other important change or Diversity Equity and Inclusion (DEI) initiatives	
Others	

Postactivity Self-reflection

1. What is my relationship with the project community?

2. How can I leverage my role, influence, and power?

3. How can I integrate this work into my day-to-day role?

WORKSHEET 4.2   Activity 2b: Clarifying Your Roles

Clarifying Your Roles Questions

1. Who is currently in charge of the change effort?

2. What roles are needed for this effort to be led effectively? (Consider the Seven Typical Change Roles handout.)

3. How will you select the best people to cover the roles you need?

Change Roles	Who will cover what roles?	How will these people be informed and introduced to the expectations of their roles?	How will you ensure that they can give their change role the attention it needs?
Sponsor			
Executive team			
Core change agent team (active cohort members)			
Change process lead			
Guiding coalition members			
Functional area (sphere) leads			
Change consultants			
Other			

4. How will you address the conflicts or time pressures for individuals who are asked to wear both a functional hat and a change role hat?

Continued

WORKSHEET 4.2   Activity 2b: Clarifying Your Roles—cont'd

5. What will you do if someone currently in the change role is not the best person for the job?

6. What consultants (internal or external) are being used in the antiracist transformation and for what purposes? How will you interface with them, integrate their activities, and bring them up to speed regarding current plans?

Postactivity Self-reflection

1. What role will you play in the change effort?

2. What strengths do you have that will help you in this role?

3. What could this role expose about you? What are your vulnerabilities you worry could limit your effectiveness?

4. What needs that, if met, would improve your ability to effectively execute your role responsibilities?

WORKSHEET 4.3   Activity 2c: Creating a Clear Case and Desired Outcome

Creating a Clear Case and Desired Outcome Discussion Questions

1. Why is the transformation needed?

2. What are the drivers of change?

3. What are the initial impacts or *big picture* outcomes on the school and its people? (Note: this is not the formal vision.)

4. Who are the target groups or those most affected by the change?

5. What is the urgency for the change? What will happen if we do not change?

Postactivity Self-reflection

1. How will you communicate the clear case and desired outcome within your sphere of influence?

2. How will you hold yourself and others accountable for communicating the case for change and the desired outcome?

WORKSHEET 4.4   Activity 2d: Creating Optical Working Relationships

Conflict Protocol Questions

1. Think about your ideal team. How would that team handle conflicts and disagreements? Jot down a few points.

2. What are some behaviors you want to have happen when conflict occurs? (For example: speak to the person directly rather than complaining behind their back, get all the stakeholders together rather than triangulating, etc.)

3. What are some things you do not want to happen when conflict occurs?

4. It takes 6 to 9 months to change behavior. How will you hold one another accountable for following these agreements? What will you or we do if someone breaks an agreement?

"Do" and "Do Not" Considerations of Conflict Protocol

Conflict protocols are useful guidelines that effective teams develop to manage conflict in a constructive way. Before developing your protocol, consider what you should do and do not do:

Do
- Be willing to resolve things without blaming.
- Get clear on why it is important to all of the parties to resolve the conflict (What is the common interest everyone has?).
- In disagreements involving multiple people, get all of the stakeholders together rather than having multiple side conversations (triangulation).
- If you have a conflict with someone, first approach them directly. If it cannot be resolved at that level, bump it up to the next level (cohort leads).
- Take responsibility for your part of the conflict. If only 2% of the complaint were true, what would that part be?
- Feed forward (the behavior change you want) rather than feedback (what someone did wrong).
- Meet your cohort agreements.
- Hold one another accountable for your agreements.

Do not
- Use team toxins (blaming, defensiveness, stonewalling, and contempt).
- Try to problem solve if someone is emotionally flooded (very upset). Take a break and come back to the conflict later.
- Triangulate (divide and conquer through multiple side conversations).
- Do hostile gossiping. If you find yourself complaining to a third party, agree to take it back to the person with whom you have a complaint.
- Practice hands from the grave. This is reopening previously agreed upon is.

Adapted from CRR Global. *About ORSC: Organization and Relationship Systems Coaching.* https://crrglobal.com/about/orsc/.

WORKSHEET 5.1   Activity 3a: Being the Change and Becoming Deeply Committed to the Change Process

Personal Daily Log

1. My Reaction Was "Centered and Effective"

Date	A. External Situation	B. Emotional Reaction	C. Physical Sensations	D. Mindset and Self-talk	E. Behaviors	F. Actions	G. Results

2. I "Reacted in a Way I Would Like to Change"

Date	A. External Situation	B. Emotional Reaction	C. Physical Sensations	D. Mindset and Self-talk	E. Behaviors	F. Actions	G. Results

Continued

WORKSHEET 5.1   Activity 3a: Being the Change and Becoming Deeply Committed to the Change Process—cont'd

Becoming the Change Questions

1. What did you learn about your way of being? Consider the patterns emerging across the columns.

2. How might your way of being influence: (1) what you see in the transformation, (2) your internal experiences with the change, (3) your decisions, (4) your impact on others, and (5) your change results or outcomes?

3. At this time, what personal transformational work might you focus on? What does that "work" look like for you?

4. How do you know when you are walking the talk of change? What are the desired behaviors, actions, and relationships?

5. What do you need, from yourself and others, in order to deeply commit to the change process?

6. How can you hold yourself accountable? What does that look like?

Postdebrief Self-reflection Questions

1. Did anything surprise you about the debrief meeting?

2. Is there anything that needs follow up or more attention at this time?

Adapted from Anderson LA, Anderson D. *The Change Leader's Roadmap: How to Navigate Your Organization's Transformation.* Vol. 384. John Wiley & Sons; 2010.

WORKSHEET 5.2 Activity 3b: Building Understanding of the Case for Change: Develop Your Initial Transformational Change Kickoff Communications

Timing	First indications of change, early stages, during design, before implementation, during implementation, postimplementation
Type of engagement	Follow instruction, offer reaction, identify impact, self-generate input, advocacy, vote/decision making, own results/implement
Level of communication	Information sharing, building understanding, identifying implications, gaining commitment, altering behavior, other
ADKAR (awareness, desire, knowledge, ability, and reinforcement) focus	Awareness, desire, knowledge, ability, reinforcement
Message content	
Delivery mechanism	
Audience/project community role	
Sender	
Status	
Notes	

WORKSHEET 5.3	Building Understanding of the Case for Change: Sponsor Roadmap
Task	
Key sponsor	
ADKAR focus	Awareness, desire, knowledge, ability, reinforcement
Priority	Low, medium, high
Support	Low, medium, high
Engagement strategy	
Due date	
Status	
Notes	

WORKSHEET 5.4   Activity 3c: Building a Powerful Enthusiastic Group of Change Leaders (Guiding Coalition): Appreciative Inquiry Interview Worksheet

Appreciative Inquiry Tool
Interviewer's Worksheet
Interviewer Name: _____
Interviewee Name: _____
Time: 40 min (20 min per interview)
Instructions:
- Take turns asking each other the following questions.
- Fill out the interview's summary worksheet after the interviewee has concluded (see below).

Interview Questions

1. What attracted you to (organization/group/field/other)?
2. What keeps you here/involved?
3. Since you joined (organization/group/field/other), you have probably experienced some ups and downs, some high points, and some low points. I would like for you to think about a high point: a time that stands out for you where you felt most effective, really proud of yourself, or really proud of your work. Please tell me the story about that time. What made it a high point experience?
4. Let us talk about some of the things you value most, specifically about yourself and about your (job/role). What are your best qualities?
5. What do you feel is the strongest, most important asset you have to offer (organization/group/field/other)?
6. What is it about (organization/group/field/other) that you value most?
7. If I could grant you three wishes for (organization/group/field/other), what would they be?

Interviewer's Summary Worksheet

What was the most quotable quote that came out of the interview?	What was the most compelling story you heard?	What two or three themes stood out for you?

Adapted from https://www.top-network.org/assets/images/monthlyfeatures/2013June/participant%20workbook%20final.pdf

WORKSHEET 5.5   Activity 3e: Building an Infrastructure and Conditions to Support Change: Communication Strategy

1. What is the vision?

2. What is my role in achieving this vision?

3. What are the obstacles preventing me from contributing to the vision?

4. Can I explain the vision and its importance to others?

5. What is the process (roadmap) for getting us to the vision?

WORKSHEET 6.1 Activity 4b: Identifying Change Targets and Developing a Tactical Plan

Description	Action Plan
TEAM. List the **MEMBERS** and their strengths/skills they can contribute to executing this tactical plan. List any other collaborators you will need.	
List your **CHANGE TARGET(S)** as concisely as you can. Make sure it includes the desired outcome or end result of your actions.	
List 3-5 **OBJECTIVES** that will be necessary to achieve your change target. Each objective should also be SMART: • Specific: includes the "who," "what," and "where." • Measurable: focuses on how much change is expected (e.g., increase or decrease) • Achievable: realistic given resources and planned implementation. • Relevant: relates directly to achieving the change target. • Time bound: focuses on when the objective will be achieved. Consider these questions when developing your objectives: • *Do your objectives support the overarching vision of your change?* • *Have you included at least one meaningful short-term objective that can be achieved quickly and that will show progress, demonstrate positive impact, and keep your sphere and others in the project community motivated to continue?* • *Are your objectives process or outcome oriented?* Process objectives describe the activities or strategies that will be used as part of achieving your change targets. Process objectives, by their nature, are usually short-term. Example: By (month/year), (X%) of faculty will be contacted (via communications and engagement opportunities) within (time period) to build buy-in and awareness of how racism is impacting our learning environment and begin to build the case for why faculty development is needed.	

Continued

WORKSHEET 6.1 Activity 4b: Identifying Change Targets and Developing a Tactical Plan—cont'd	
Outcome objectives specify the intended effect of the change target or end result. The outcome objectives focus on what your project community will know or be able to do as a result of the change target. Example: By (month/year), faculty who attended (x training sessions) will demonstrate an increase in anti-racist practices during lectures and small group sessions.	
RESOURCES	
CHALLENGES	
SUCCESS FACTORS Identify factors needed to ensure your tactical plan will be successfully implemented.	
Notes:	

WORKSHEET 6.2   Activity 4c: Setting up an Accountability and Outcome Tracking System: Results-Based Accountability

Sphere/group: _____

Date: _____

Instructions

1. Select one of our *change targets*:
2. Identify *change target stakeholder*(s):
3. What is the goal or end result of the change target?
4. Consider our work to date or upcoming work towards our change target. In the following box, complete each quadrant by answering the questions in the box:

Quantity How much did we do? (Q1) How will we track how much we deliver or implement? (Consider number of attendees, number of activities, etc.)	**Quality** How well did we do it? (Q2) How will we track the quality of our deliverables or actions we implemented? (Consider percentage of activities performed well, feedback from stakeholders, etc.)

Effect

Is anyone better off? (Q3)

How can we begin to track the impact of the change we produce? Ask "In what ways is the stakeholder group in our project community better off as a result of our efforts? How would we know, in measurable terms, if they were better off?"

This is more difficult to determine and might require monitoring change over time. Create pairs of measures (number and percent) for each answer.

(Consider number/percentage with improvement in behaviors, attitudes, or skills.)

Number of behaviors, attitudes, or skill	Percentage behavior, attitudes, or skill

5. In Q2 and Q3, circle or highlight the measures for which we have good data.
6. Review the list of brainstormed performance measures that we have not circled or highlighted. List the top performance measures that we would like to develop data for and track (i.e., what can "tell the story" of our change and impact):
   a.
   b.
   c.
7. Now what? What are the next steps?

Friedman M. *Trying Hard Is Not Good Enough: How to Produce Measurable Improvements for Customers and Communities.* 10th Anniversary ed. KDPamazon; 2015.

WORKSHEET 6.3 **Activity 4e: Designing a Proactive Resistance Management Plan: Resistance Management Plan**	
Impacted group/ project community role	Based on existing evidence, which group or project community role or stakeholder might be resistant to the antiracist change?
ADKAR barrier(s)	Awareness: Desire: Knowledge: Ability: Reinforcement:
Resistance anticipated or identified	What type of resistance and when do you think it might emerge?
How to identify resistance	What will the resistance look or sound like? Name the behaviors.
Approach for managing resistance	What is the approach? Who will take on what actions?

Prosci. *Managing Resistance to Change Overview.* https://www.prosci.com/resources/articles/managing-resistance-to-change.

WORKSHEET 6.4 Activity 4g: Developing a Communication Plan: Engagement and Communication Plan

Timing	First indications of change, early stages, during design, before implementation, during implementation, postimplementation
Type of engagement	Follow instruction, offer reaction, identify impact, self-generate input, advocacy, vote/decision making, own results/implement
Level of Communication	Information sharing, building understanding, identifying implications, gaining commitment, altering behavior, other
ADKAR focus	Awareness, desire, knowledge, ability, reinforcement
Message content	
Delivery mechanism	
Audience/project community role	
Sender	
Status	
Notes:	

WORKSHEET 7.1 Activity 5a: Embracing Emergence: Dialogue

Reminder: We recommend the guiding coalition periodically revisit the dialogue and worksheet as needed.

1. Small is good, small is all – the large is a reflection of the small.

As a guiding coalition, how can we keep an eye on what is happening on a small scale, not just large-scale actions or big wins?

2. Change is constant – "Be like water."

As a guiding coalition, how can we prevent ourselves from being restricted or trapped by our mindset and approach?
How can we adapt to certain situations, grow, and change as the transformation unfolds?
What are the ways in which we can pay attention to what is happening within our group (with each other) and with the project community?
How can we empower ourselves to invent, experiment, create, and learn?
What strategies can we imagine that respect the changing nature of change itself?

3. There is always enough time for the "right" work.

As a guiding coalition, how can we go where there is energy?
How can we be attuned and pay attention to what is trying to emerge?

4. Never a failure, always a lesson.

As a guiding coalition, how can we turn breakdowns into breakthroughs?
What mental models and behaviors must we use to help us examine and learn from our failures?
How can we create brave spaces to do this?

5. Trust the people – if you trust the people, they become trustworthy.

As a guiding coalition, in what ways can we trust each other and those involved in the change?
What will this look and feel like?

WORKSHEET 7.1   Activity 5a: Embracing Emergence: Dialogue—cont'd

6. Move at the speed of trust.

As a guiding coalition, what are the ways in which we are vulnerable and authentic?
What are the ways in which our change target strategies include building trust to accelerate the change?

---

7. Focus on critical connections more than critical mass – build resilience by building relationships.

As a guiding coalition, what are the ways in which we are actively building relationships with each other and those involved in the change?

---

8. Less prep, more presence.

As a guiding coalition, what are the ways in which we can hold ourselves accountable for shifting from preparing to being present?
How will we know when we are being present?
How can we ensure we are not always on autopilot or relying on the plan to drive our actions?

---

9. What you pay attention to, grows.

As the transformation emerges, how can we as a guiding coalition balance critique with having an appreciation for what is good and strength based?
In what ways can we identify and focus on positive energy throughout the change?

Brown AM. *Emergent Strategy: Shaping Change, Changing Worlds*. Ak Press; 2017.

WORKSHEET 7.2   Activity 5b: Learning and Course Correcting

Incentive, Risk, and Burden

Incentive	What is our incentive for using a course correction process in our transformation? What are the benefits?
Risk	What is the risk of not using a course correction process?
Burden	What is the burden to the guiding coalition, sponsor(s), change strategy team, and the project community of using a course correction process?

Building Your Course Correction System

Content. Identify what will require feedback. Consider your change targets and plans.

Sources. Identify the most likely sources of feedback: who might have feedback or input? Review the project community for key people and groups who must be informed about and involved in generating input to the course correction process.

Vehicles. Identify the vehicles that will be used for gathering data and feedback. Weigh the pros and cons of face-to-face (meetings, conversations, focus groups, listening circles, brown bag lunches, etc.), and the use of technology (video conferencing, phone, website, email, newsletter, Teams, etc.).

Person responsible. Identify the point person or place for people to bring feedback, aberrant data, or wake-up calls about the change.

WORKSHEET 7.2   Activity 5b: Learning and Course Correcting—cont'd

Using new information. Clarify your process for dealing with and deciding how to use feedback and new information to correct either the outcomes of your change or how it is being implemented.

Communicating back. Determine how you will communicate the impact of feedback or new information, whether it was used, and how it caused things to evolve. With whom do you need to communicate? Think about the people or groups who generated this input.

Resources. What resources are required to support your course correction system, and how will you obtain them? Might you need, for instance, budget, meeting space, or technology?

Announcement. Determine how you will communicate to your project community and/or institution about your system, and how it is being used.

Consider the Change Sponsor(s) and Leaders

Identify how to gain agreement among the sponsor(s) and leaders about the importance of learning and course correction in leading the transformational change.

Why it is essential to the new antiracist culture of the institution?

Anderson LA, Anderson D. *The Change Leader's Roadmap: How to Navigate Your Organization's Transformation.* Vol. 384. John Wiley & Sons; 2010.

WORKSHEET 7.3 Activity 5c: Monitoring Progress Markers and Strategy: Outcome Journal

1. Record the "outcome challenge" for each stakeholder group.
Briefly describe the behaviors, relationships, activities, and actions of individuals, or groups that will change if you were successful at promoting readiness to change?

2. Identify the progress markers for each stakeholder group.
Identify the progress markers for each stakeholder group: • Expect to see = change in behavior relatively easy to achieve. • Like to see = change in behavior that indicates active learning or engagement. • Love to see = change in behavior that is transformative.

Stakeholder Group	*Expect* to See	*Like* to See	*Love* to See

—— Monitoring (Post Session) ——

3. Provide a brief description of change.

4. Identify the contributing factors and actions.

WORKSHEET 7.3 Activity 5c: Monitoring Progress Markers and Strategy: Outcome Journal—cont'd

5. List the source of evidence.

6. Report on any unanticipated change.

7. Identify lessons and required changes or reactions.

Earl S, Carden F, Patton MQ, Smutylo T, International Development Research Centre (Canada). *Outcome Mapping: Building Learning and Reflection into Development Programs.* Inter national Development Research Centre; 2001.

WORKSHEET 7.4 Activity 5c: Monitoring Progress Markers and Strategy: Strategy Journal

DESCRIPTION OF ACTIVITIES			EFFECTIVENESS
What did you do?	With whom?	When?	How did it influence change with stakeholders?
Strategy 1:			
Strategy 2:			
Strategy 3:			
Lessons and Required Changes or Follow-up Add more to the list as needed ... 1. 2. 3.			

Earl S, Carden F, Patton MQ, Smutylo T, International Development Research Centre (Canada). *Outcome Mapping: Building Learning and Reflection into Development Programs*. Inte rnational Development Research Centre; 2001.

WORKSHEET 7.5   Activity 5d: Reacting to Resistance: Resistance Management

Identifying the Root Causes of the Resistance

What's one word to describe how you feel about recent changes?

What's working for you or your group right now? What's not? Why do you think that is?

What are your hopes? What are your fears? Where do those feelings come from?

What do you need in order to be successful?

Corrective Actions - ADKAR

If **awareness** was the root cause, examine past communications and messages to the individual or group. Create messages that address any gaps in building awareness of why the change is needed. Do you need to reiterate the case for change?

If **desire** was the root cause, assess the incentives or consequences that would create motivation to change. Are these incentives or consequences sufficient? Do adjustments to the incentives or consequences need to be made? Are these incentives and consequences understood?

Continued

WORKSHEET 7.5   Activity 5d: Reacting to Resistance: Resistance Management—cont'd

If **knowledge** was the root cause, examine the opportunities for the project community to learn more about how to change. Assess the attendance and effectiveness of these learning opportunities. Is additional education needed? Do current offerings need to be redesigned? Are there gaps in the knowledge and skills being taught?

If **ability** was the root cause, personal assistance may be required. What timely assistance is being offered?

If **reinforcement** was the root cause, what systems, values or reward systems reinforce the change?

Activate Roles to Manage Resistance

On an ongoing basis, are the senior leaders actively and visibly reinforcing the case for change?

What are the ways in which the senior leaders can help manage the resistance in other ways?

Who will help coach the senior leaders on their role?

Inc., P. The PROSCI ADKAR® model, Prosci. Available at https://www.prosci.com/methodology/adkar.[9]

WORKSHEET 7.6 Activity 5e: Supporting Integration and Mastery: Integration and Mastery

What strategies will you use to support individuals and teams to uncover how they can master their part of the new state?
What are the ways in which you will identify and reinforce integration over time?
How will you handle this work with dispersed, hybrid, or virtual teams?
How will you ensure that individuals and teams consciously model the new mindsets, behaviors, culture, and relationships after the launch or "go live" of your change targets?
How will you make the case to the sponsor(s) to invest in a "whole system" integration and mastery process?

Anderson LA, Anderson D. *The Change Leader's Roadmap: How to Navigate Your Organization's Transformation.* Vol. 384. John Wiley & Sons; 2010.

WORKSHEET 7.7   Activity 5f: Celebrating the Achievements: Creating Celebrations

What methods will you use to celebrate and reward people's efforts to create the new state?

How can you use your communications and celebrations to further reinforce the mindset, values, norms, and behaviors required for the success of the new antiracist state?

How will you ensure that the project community understands the need for further changes?

How can you reinforce the notion that antiracism is an ongoing process that requires celebration of small wins along the journey?

Anderson LA, Anderson D. *The Change Leader's Roadmap: How to Navigate Your Organization's Transformation.* Vol. 384. John Wiley & Sons; 2010; Prosci. *The Prosci ADKAR Model.* https://www.prosci.com/methodology/adkar.

WORKSHEET 7.8   Activity 5g: Removing Barriers: Removing Barriers

Why is this considered a barrier?

What impact would it have on the change effort and change targets?

What could the guiding coalition, change strategy team, and sponsor do about it? What would be most effective?

When should this be done?

Who should lead what actions or efforts to remove the barriers? Who is responsible or accountable?

INDEX